Learning to care on the PAEDIATRIC WARD

Helen Lewer
BSc (Hons), RGN, RSCN, RNT

Senior Nurse: Tutor, Paediatrics and
Nursing Practice, The Nightingale School,
St Thomas' Hospital, London

Edward Arnold
A division of Hodder & Stoughton
LONDON BALTIMORE MELBOURNE AUCKLAND

LEARNING TO CARE SERIES

General Editors

JEAN HEATH, MED, BA, SRN, SCM, CERT ED
English National Board Learning Resources Unit, Sheffield

SUSAN E NORMAN, SRN, DNCERT, RNT
Formerly Senior Tutor, The Nightingale School, West Lambeth Health Authority

First published in Great Britain 1988

British Library Cataloguing in Publication Data

Lewer, Helen
Learning to care on the paediatric ward
1. Hospitals. Patients: Children – For nursing
I. Title
610.73'62

ISBN 0-340-41175-9

Typeset in 10/11 pt Trump Medieval by
Rowland Phototypesetting Ltd, Bury St Edmunds, Suffolk

Printed and bound in Great Britain for Edward Arnold, the educational, academic and medical publishing division of Hodder & Stoughton Ltd, 41 Bedford Square, London WC1B 3DP by Richard Clay Ltd, Bungay, Suffolk

CONTENTS

EDITORS' FOREWORD

In most professions there is a traditional gulf between theory and its practice, and nursing is no exception. The gulf is perpetuated when theory is taught in a theoretical setting and practice is taught by the practitioner.

This inherent gulf has to be bridged by students of nursing, and publication of this series is an attempt to aid such bridge building.

It aims to help relate theory and practice in a meaningful way whilst underlining the importance of the person being cared for.

It aims to introduce students of nursing to some of the more common problems found in each new area of experience in which they will be asked to work.

It aims to de-mystify some of the technical language they will hear, putting it in context, giving it meaning and enabling understanding.

PREFACE

Children today are likely to be faced with many stresses and strains, arising from changes in society. It is therefore important, that when they are sick, children be nursed within an environment which they know and by people with whom they are familiar. The ideal place for most children to be is at home, wherever that home may be. However, it is not always possible to nurse the child there and admission to hospital becomes necessary, often urgent, as the condition of a sick child can deteriorate rapidly.

Paediatric wards aim to make the transition from home to hospital less traumatic for the child and family, who are already likely to be anxious. Part of the transition is encouraging the family to be resident or visit freely, participating in their child's care whenever they wish to do so. Family involvement in care makes the role of the nurse in paediatrics very different from other areas of nursing. Not only is the nurse working with the child, but also with the family. The role becomes one of facilitator of care and care giver – a partnership between family and nurse. This role is not always easy and students allocated to the paediatric ward need time and the appropriate support to adjust.

Learners who may be working in the paediatric ward include those on an RGN or EN(G) programme and, in the near future, learners undertaking conversion courses. This book is aimed at providing the necessary background knowledge which these groups of students need to nurse sick children. It may also be useful as a 'refresher' for those commencing the RSCN course, or for mature candidates returning to nursing. The content is more detailed than some introductory paediatric texts – this is intentional as nursing children requires a new and wide range of knowledge and skills. It is also detailed care, drawing from the appropriate knowledge in the biopsychosocial and nursing sciences.

The book is organised around a nursing framework, that of the Activities of Living (Roper *et al.* 1985), with chapter headings reflecting the activity to be considered. One of the principles of Roper's model is dependence–independence and this links with the developmental processes of childhood. Case histories are included to 'set the scene' for nursing care which is shown using detailed care plans. The practical application of the nursing process is included to guide learners with planning individualised care when in the paediatric ward. Learners are invited to complete various exercises, shown at intervals during the text. The child is considered whilst in hospital and the book does not attempt to include more than background details of community care.

Nursing children requires special knowledge and skills, a fact noted in the Ministry of Health 1959 Platt report, but still not fully implemented in 1988.

Children are a challenge to nurse, but the rewards are enormous.

ACKNOWLEDGEMENTS

To Robert and my family for their support and encouragement. To Ursula Cowell, Director of Nurse Education, The Nightingale School, for her advice. To Graham – my critic! – and to the November 1986 students who read and criticised the text. Finally to Barbara Phillips for her professional typing and presentation of the manuscript.

1 An introduction to paediatric care

Caring for children can be stimulating and rewarding and is an experience which many students look forward to in the RGN programme.

This text discusses children in their home or community setting as well as when they are in hospital. Consideration of children within their normal surroundings must be included in all aspects of their care in hospital. Children will usually return to the same environment and way of life after hospitalisation and therefore this transitional period of care can be influential and important to their future.

HOME OR HOSPITAL?

Ideally, when children are ill they should be nursed at home, with their family around them. However, sometimes the family cannot cope due to environmental, social or employment constraints or because the child becomes too ill to be nursed at home. Parents often feel they have failed in their care when a child needs hospitalisation and it is quite difficult for them to visit either the general practitioner (GP) or a casualty department. At other times, enormous relief is felt when medical and nursing attention can be given quickly. Parents need not be separated from their children and this principle should be remembered in all aspects of care and treatment.

A link with the community can be maintained through the liaison health visitor, family health visitor, GP or clinical nurse specialists. Too often these links are tenuous, but they can be very supportive especially where long-term illness or other problems are present.

Cultural and ethnic differences

Careful attention should be paid to cultural and ethnic differences in families whose child is admitted to hospital. This may affect who cares for the child and how visiting is arranged. It may affect how the child eats and drinks, as well as communicates, cleanses, dresses and eliminates. Families with specific cultural backgrounds often have particular spiritual needs.

Why children are admitted to hospital

The reasons why children need to be admitted to hospital include the whole range of illnesses noted in the adult lifespan, as well as all those which are related to childhood. The nurse in the paediatric ward can expect to nurse a wide range of illness. Below is an arbitrary grouping of some illnesses using the 12 Activities of Living (Roper *et al.* 1985) which require admission of children to hospital (some appear in more than one category).

Lack of a safe environment
- Infections and infectious diseases* (e.g. meningitis; eye infections)
- Trauma (e.g. fractures; burns*)
- Ingestion or inhalation
- Child abuse
- Social reasons

Failure of effective communication
- Speech, hearing or sight defects, also mental retardation
- Congenital deformities (e.g. cleft lip and palate)

* Topics given further consideration in subsequent chapters.

Behaviour problems
Chromosomal abnormalities (e.g. Down's Syndrome)
Social reasons

Breathing and circulatory problems
Genetic deformities (e.g. sickle cell anaemia*; haemophilia; cystic fibrosis)
Congenital heart defects
Allergic conditions (e.g. asthma)
Infections (e.g. croup*; bronchiolitis)

Difficulties associated with maintaining a constant body temperature
Infections (e.g. meningitis; febrile convulsions*)

Difficulties with eating and drinking
Congenital deformities (e.g. pyloric stenosis*)
Dietary and malabsorption problems (e.g. obesity*; failure to thrive – coeliac disease and cystic fibrosis)
Infections (e.g. gastroenteritis)
Intestinal obstruction
Social reasons

Problems with eliminating and personal cleansing and dressing
Anatomical deformities and developmental problems (e.g. constipation)
Neoplasia (e.g. Wilms' tumour)
Infections (e.g. infected eczema; gastroenteritis)
Social reasons (e.g. constipation*; head lice*)

Difficulty in mobilising, working, playing and sleeping
Trauma (e.g. fractures)
Congenital defects caused at birth (e.g. spina bifida; cerebral palsy*)
Developmental problems
Social reasons

Problems associated with normal sexuality
Changes to body image (e.g. burns*)
Safety and social reasons (e.g. sexual abuse*)

Cause of death
Neoplasia (e.g. leukaemia)
Prematurity
Congenital deformities

Children admitted for planned* or emergency* surgery make up a large number of admissions to the paediatric ward. Examples of planned surgery include tonsillectomies, herniorrhaphy* and circumcision. For emergency surgery, children admitted for removal of foreign bodies in the airway, appendicectomies and so on.

Where children are nursed in hospital

Puberty heralds the onset of adolescence, with changes in general and sexual body characteristics. Children who have not reached this phase are **prepubertal**.

Children who are prepubertal should be nursed in a paediatric ward. In 1959, the Platt Report advocated that this was the most suitable place for children to be nursed. A report in 1987 by the National Association for the Welfare of Children in Hospital (NAWCH) shows that while the situation is better than at the time of the Platt recommendations, children are still being nursed in adult wards. This can have a serious effect on the child, as well as often hindering free visiting and residency by parents and preventing access to the specialist skills of paediatric nursing and medical staff.

Infants who require treatment at birth are usually nursed in a Special Care Baby Unit (SCBU) which may be run by either midwifery or paediatric staff.

When emergency or specialist treatment is necessary infants may be transferred to a paediatric hospital. This can be a very upsetting time for new parents, especially the child's mother who has to remain behind in the hospital midwifery department. Photographs taken of the infant can be a very useful link at such a time.

From infancy to adolescence, children should be nursed in a paediatric ward either in a District General Hospital, or in a private hospital, or when specialist care is needed, in a regional paediatric centre.

Where possible, adolescents should be nursed in their own unit, however there are very few adolescent units in the UK. An adolescent is usually placed in a paediatric or an adult ward, this being determined by the medical team on admission.

If children become extremely ill they may be transferred to an Intensive Care Unit (ITU) in their own hospital. This is not an ideal situation and where possible they should be transferred to a specialist paediatric ITU. However, the trauma of being nursed in an ITU can be lessened by encouraging parents to visit freely, be resident and participate in the child's care. Treatment should be given by paediatricians and surgeons and nursing care by trained paediatric nurses (RSCNs).

Other places where children may be nursed and cared for are psychiatric day hospitals, renal units and children's homes.

A mention should be made of the benefit of having day care facilities for toddlers, preschoolers and for children not needing a lengthy period of hospitalisation. Many paediatric units have a ward or part of a ward for this.

Who should nurse children?

First and foremost, the family should nurse children if they are willing and capable of doing so. The role of the nurse is often to advise or supervise as well as to give expert nursing care. In the USA and in some places in the UK, parent-care units have been set up. Parents are not left alone to cope but they are able to give most of the care for their child during the period of hospitalisation. This has to be carefully negotiated with the nursing staff, who sometimes consider their role as one of 'mother substitute' for children in hospital. Parents can be amazing in accomplishing numerous technical procedures. Parenteral nutrition, stoma care and giving injections are just some of the things parents will undertake in hospital and at home. The underlying principle here is to teach and support the parents so that they feel able to cope.

The nursing staff who care for children should be Registered Sick Children's Nurses (RSCNs). At the present time, this qualification is not mandatory for those applying to work in paediatrics. There are unique and specialist skills associated with nursing sick children, as well as the understanding of developmental changes in childhood, which an RSCN course teaches.

The concept of giving expert care has to be balanced by the ability to work with parents in sharing care of their child. It can be quite difficult at first for nurses new to the paediatric ward to see the benefit of having parents, siblings and relatives around much of the time. It is even more difficult where the parents, who may be the same age as the nurse, turn to her for advice. But families should be welcomed and catered for at all times in the paediatric ward. (See Chapter 11 for some thoughts on the future of paediatric nursing.)

The ages and stages of childhood

The different ages and stages of childhood are defined generally, as well as in this text, so that biopsychosocial changes can be related to specific age groups. Often the key changes which happen at each stage of development are called 'milestones', or stepping stones.

In this text and throughout every chapter which considers an activity of living, the following stages of childhood development have been used.

Infants	0–1 year
Toddlers	1–2½ years
Preschool children	2½–5 years
School children	5–11 years
Adolescents	11–18 years

Using individual care and the nursing process in paediatrics

The individual care approach to children supports the concept of holism, where the child is considered as an individual within a family and community setting. It is virtually impossible to nurse one part of the child (e.g. a fractured leg) without considering the effect this will have on the rest of his body, his mind and his family.

In this text, examples of care plans have been given and the terminology used for the care plan is as follows:

Care plan terminology
Nursing history and assessment of normal routines
Identification of problems in order of priority
Goals
Nursing action and rationale
Evaluation

Together with individual care, the logical and systematic approach offered by the nursing process is ideal when applied to paediatric nursing.

The need to assess the child, his family and his community background (environment, social and other factors) constitutes the basis of a problem-solving approach, whilst setting the child within the context of his 'normal' routine. In finding out about the child, safer care should be offered. The goal setting, actioning and evaluating of care completes the nursing process cycle and allows for the changes and flexibility which must be incorporated when nursing children.

Because of the intimate nature of this type of nursing, confidentiality must be maintained (see UKCC *Code of Professional Conduct* 1984). One other consideration is that the more involved the nurse becomes with the child and his parents, the more difficult it may become for her to break the relationship when the child goes home, or in sadder circumstances, dies. The stress associated with using an individualised approach to caring for children should be a point for discussion.

Using the Activities of Living

The Activities of Living framework as described by Roper *et al.* (1985) lends itself not only to the individual child, but also to consideration of the developmental changes of childhood. This text is arranged in chapters using the 12 Activities of Living to explore development in each activity to a greater depth.

Another reason why this framework is appropriate for paediatric nursing is that it supports the health–illness continuum. As children progress along the lifespan continuum, they also develop biopsychosocially and this helps towards gaining independence. When considering the activities, one should acknowledge the concepts underpinning this model which are health–illness, dependence–independence and the life cycle.

Roper *et al.* (1985) illustrate this clearly when they chart the development in all the activities of a 5-year-old child.

Fig. 1.1 Dependence–independence continuum related to the 12 Activities of Living (based on Roper *et al.* 1985)

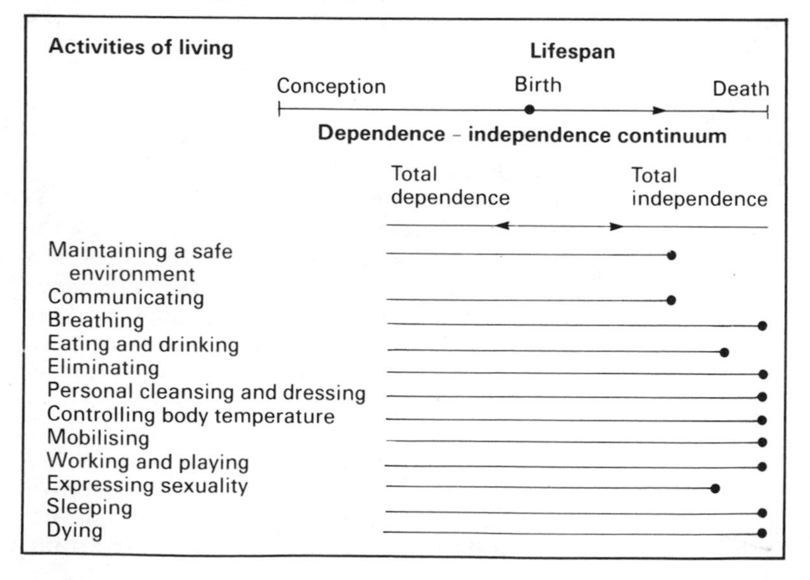

EXERCISE

Using the same framework (Fig. 1.2), attempt to plot the development of a normal 2-year-old child on the figure below. You may find it helpful to read this book through first.

Fig. 1.2 Exercise to plot a dependence–independence continuum for a normal 2-year-old child

	Total dependence	Total independence
Maintaining a safe environment		
Communicating		
Breathing		
Eating and drinking		
Eliminating		
Personal cleansing and dressing		
Controlling body temperature		
Mobilising		
Working and playing		
Expressing sexuality		
Sleeping		
Dying		

Although Roper *et al.* (1985) do not specifically state that their model promotes self-care, by virtue of encouraging independence and in relation to the development of the skills in physical, mental and social fields, this should assist the child in becoming self-caring. The model can also encourage a health educative approach.

Each of the 12 activities is an observable feature of living, hence the terminology. For example, 'breathing' is written as an action-based activity. Dying is the last observable activity of any human being. It should also be remembered that each activity encompasses biological, psychosocial, environmental, cultural, and politico-economic factors. An

Table 1.1 An example of a 2-year-old child's normal routine which might be obtained when taking a nursing history/assessment when the child is admitted to hospital, and using the 12 Activities of Living. (A nursing history sheet is shown in full in Chapter 2)

ADMISSION TO HOSPITAL		
ACTIVITY	NORMAL ROUTINE	PROBLEM
Maintaining a safe environment	Goes up, but can fall over coming downstairs. Still overbalances at times, when running. Supervision needed with all activities. Completed the infant/toddler immunisation programme.	
Communicating	250 words spoken, using simple short sentences. Points to objects wanted. Gets cross when stopped from being independent – stamps feet and cries. Verbalises pain ('hurts'). Junior analgesia given. Won't be parted from mother for long.	
Breathing	Pulse: 110 beats/min Respirations: 20–30/min Blood pressure: 95/61 mmHg Blocked nose and irritating cough when a cold is present. Skin colour healthy.	
Eating and drinking	Eats adult foods, cut up, small amounts, no salt and a balanced diet. Feeds self with a spoon and drinks from a cup (tea, milk, juices etc.) Wears a plastic bib. Weight: 12.6 kg	
Eliminating	Potty training in progress. Nappies at night. Urinates: 6 times a day. Defaecates: once a day.	
Personal cleansing and dressing	Supervision with washing. Cleans teeth with a soft toothbrush. Brushes hair. Puts on main items of clothing, but needs help especially with buttons, laces and ties.	
Controlling body temperature	T: 37°C Pyrexia when infection present.	

ADMISSION TO HOSPITAL		
ACTIVITY	NORMAL ROUTINE	PROBLEM
	No febrile convulsions. Gets cold hands and feet.	
Mobilising	Runs, jumps, rides a plastic trike. Mobilises without thought for own safety. Height: 85 cm (see weight also for centile chart)	
Working and playing	Toddler group with mother, three times a week. Has own toys, doesn't share. Special toy is a cuddly bear.	
Expressing sexuality	Becoming interested in body parts and genitals.	
Sleeping	Sleeps 6p.m. – 6a.m. One hour nap after lunch. Used to sleeping in a room with brother. Needs to be lifted at 10p.m. for a dry night.	
Dying	No comprehension of death. Dislikes upset to routine, so saves grandad a place at the table.	

example of this may be seen in relation to eating and drinking. A Hindu child, whilst not being affected physically or psychosocially by eating, may in fact be used to sitting on the floor to eat, with his family, not eating beef or pork and only eating one bowl of food once a day.

Although spiritual activities are not assessed as a separate activity of living (whereas Henderson (1966) states this is a human need) their influence on any activity must be taken into account.

USING THE TEXT

The chapter you have been reading introduces the concept of child care in hospital, using the Activities of Living framework in planning individualised care.

Chapters 2 and 3 concentrate on safety and

communication and together with this chapter provide the basis for paediatric care and for the subsequent chapters in the book. Chapters 4–10 discuss the other activities of living as they affect children across the developmental stages. In some instances (i.e. Chapter 7) elimination is described in conjunction with personal cleansing and dressing. Although each activity is considered individually, each should be read as contributing to the child as a whole.

Features included in each chapter are as follows:

- health promotion and education in relation to stages of development;
- related anatomy and physiology;
- patient histories and care plans, including education and aftercare of the child and family; and
- topical subjects (e.g. child abuse).

These may be series of questions, identifying problems for the care plan or completing a care plan. Other exercises include medicine calculations and finding out about the care and treatment of specific illnesses.

REFERENCES

HENDERSON, V. 1966. *The Nature of Nursing.* Collier Macmillan, London.

MINISTRY OF HEALTH 1959. *The Welfare of Children in Hospital,* Report of the Platt Committee. HMSO, London.

NATIONAL ASSOCIATION FOR THE WELFARE OF CHILDREN IN HOSPITALS. 1987. *Where are the Children?* Report of the Caring for Children in the Health Services Joint Committee (RCN, NAHA, BPA & NAWCH), London.

ROPER, N., LOGAN, W. & TIERNEY, A. J. 1985. *The Elements of Nursing,* 2nd Edn. Churchill Livingstone, Edinburgh.

UNITED KINGDOM CENTRAL COUNCIL. 1984. *Code of Professional Conduct for the Nurse, Midwife and Health Visitor,* 2nd Edn. UKCC, London.

FURTHER READING

CLEARY, J. 1977. The distribution of nursing attention in a children's ward. *Nursing Times*, **73** (28).

ENGLISH NATIONAL BOARD. 1985. *Caring for Children. A workbook for nurses in general training*. ENB, London.

Fit for the future. 1976. Report of the court committee. HMSO, London.

JOLLY, J. 1981. *The other side of paediatrics: A guide to the everyday care of sick children*. Macmillan, London.

KALUGER, G. & KALUGER, M. F. 1979. *Human Development. The span of life*, 2nd Edn. Mosby, London.

PILL, R. 1977. The long stay child patient: The problems. *Nursing Times*, **73**(27), 89–92.

STACEY, M. 1970. *Hospitals, Children and Families*. Routledge & Kegan Paul, London.

THE NATIONAL BOARDS FOR ENGLAND AND WALES. 1985. *Aspects of sick children's nursing. A learning package*. The National Boards, London and Cardiff.

2 Maintaining a safe environment

SAFETY

Safety of the environment, both at home and in hospital, must be one of the main concepts underlying childcare. The need for vigilance in everything that children do cannot be stressed enough.

By nature, children are inquisitive and explore their environment in order to learn and develop. Safety is usually of great concern to parents and includes such aspects as feed preparation, safe handling, safe toys, equipment and the household environment.

Safety can also be considered in relation to protecting the child from infection, trauma or any illness.

To illustrate maintenance of safety in the paediatric ward, the following examples are included:

1 Isolation nursing – an exercise comprises part of this section;
2 Pre- and post-operative care using the first three activities of living to structure the care plans;
3 Calculations of medicines exercise; and
4 Child abuse – failure of safe care.

Health promotion and education

Although the onus is on parents to provide a safe environment, other personnel and facilities are available to give advice.

At birth, infants are registered on the Register of Births, Marriages and Deaths. This provides statistics about mortality and allows the family to claim benefits and welfare.

The midwife is the first person the family may encounter for advice after the birth of their child. The midwife and GP are likely to have been involved with the antenatal care of the mother. The midwife, whether at home or in hospital, checks the child's initial development (see Chapter 8, Mobilising, working playing and sleeping). She may also give advice on feeding, warmth and handling of the infant, as well as community and welfare provisions. Screening is carried out for phenylketonuria by the Guthrie test and for hypothyroidism (cretinism).

In hospital a physical examination will have been performed to establish if congenital dislocation of the hip is present. A general assessment of development is made (including measurements) to establish the infant's potential to develop normally.

After 10 days the health visitor takes over the care of the family. The health visitor's role is to advise on and promote child health, until the age of five years, when the child starts school. This will include advice about safety, as well as feeding, clothing, equipment, toys and immunisations. Developmental assessments begin at six weeks and continue at regular intervals until five years (refer to Chapter 8, Mobilising, working, playing and sleeping). Pamphlets, magazines, newspapers and other sections of the media all offer advice on health and safety matters for parents.

The family GP has a commitment to care for the child throughout life, but is usually involved only when illness occurs, although some GPs like to perform the developmental assessments and give immunisations.

During preschool and school years, children develop outdoor play and campaigns concerned with road and play safety are aimed at young children, as well as at parents and teachers. The Royal Society for the Prevention of Accidents (RoSPA) visit schools to give talks and often provide courses, such as safe cycling. Children are curious to know more about safety in general, but particularly road and water safety (Moon 1987).

The school medical team visits the school at regular intervals to assess the child's development and to identify any children needing referral or treatment. The school nurse is a key worker in this team as she may spend more time on site with the children and therefore should have a health educative role (see Hanson 1987).

By adolescence, the emphasis for safety is on self-care. The adolescent is liable to experiment, which may be detrimental to health. Campaigns about smoking, alcohol, drug abuse and sex and associated diseases are aimed at teenagers to prevent them damaging their health and future.

Safety factors at different developmental stages

The infant 0–1 years

During the first year of life, there is little if any comprehension of safety. When safety fails, the infant may be hurt physically or psychologically. Pain may be a learning factor for the infant for future experiences.

Correct handling and positioning of the infant

(Refer also to Chapter 8, Mobilising, working, playing and sleeping.)

Because the infant's body is disproportionate in head to body ratio, the head must always be supported whenever he is lifted or moved.

Table 2.1 Accident types in the under fives. The Department of Trade and Industry's Home Accident Surveillance System (HASS) estimated that in 1986 under fives suffered 485 000 accidents (24% of all accidents) (Data from Department of Trade and Industry, 1987)

ACCIDENT TYPE	APPROXIMATE PERCENTAGE OF TOTAL ACCIDENTS IN THE UNDER FIVES
Unknown	6%
Other	3%
Poisoning/inhalation	8%
Foreign body	7%
Burn	6%
Cut/pierce	7%
Struck	17%
Falls	46%

The infant also responds well to firm and secure handling especially at bath and feed times, when being weighed or played with.

Positioning the infant in the cot or pram should take account of susceptibility to inhale milk or secretions (refer to Chapter 4, Breathing).

Provision of a constant temperature

(Refer to Chapter 5, Maintaining body temperature)

Immature development of the temperature-regulating mechanisms and inability to control his own environment, predispose the infant to extremes of body temperature.

Protection from infection

The infant has a primitive immune system with some passive immunity being acquired from the mother during foetal life. As the infant comes into contact with differing antigens he develops his own antibodies. Immunisations are given to provide immunity against diseases which can be harmful to the infant if contracted naturally (e.g. diphtheria and whooping cough).

Parents are advised not to place infants in contact with crowds of people, or indeed those suffering from infectious diseases. In families with brothers and sisters the contact may be unavoidable.

With the ever-increasing problem of AIDS and HIV-positive adults, infants who are also positive for the human immunodeficiency virus acquired through parents or through breast milk, are a growing concern for all personnel concerned with infant and child care. Children who inherit the defect causing haemophilia have been at risk from receiving infected blood products, but should now be more protected as all blood donors are screened for the human immunodeficiency viruses.

Table 2.2 An immunisation programme

AGE	TYPE OF IMMUNISATION
Up to 3 months	No immunisations given. Smallpox or tuberculosis (TB) can be given if there is contact with an infected person or if a country is to be visited where smallpox or tuberculosis are present.
At 3–4 months 7–8 months	Diphtheria, pertussis and tetanus (DPT triple vaccine) and poliomyelitis oral vaccine.
At 15 months	Measles vaccine. At least six weeks after the last triple or polio vaccination. Recently measles, mumps and rubella vaccine.
3–3½ years	Preschool booster dose of diphtheria and tetanus vaccine. Poliomyelitis booster dose.
11–12 years	Rubella vaccine for girls (for the present).
12–14 years	BCG vaccination against tuberculosis if Mantoux-negative.

Note: Criteria for the DPT and polio schedule should be one month between the first and second dose. Double vaccine (diphtheria and tetanus) is available and may be recommended where there is a history of convulsions or developmental or neurological defects in the child.
Poliomyelitis is contra-indicated in children hypersensitive to penicillin.

There are many individual factors to be considered for children before immunisation is given, and the GP or health visitor should take a careful history from each family. See *Immunisation against infectious diseases* (DHSS, 1984).

Provision of sterile and correctly diluted feeds

(Refer to Chapter 6, Eating and drinking.)

Feeds and feeding equipment must be sterile for infants up to one year.

Provision of safe playthings

(Refer to Chapter 8, Mobilising, working, playing and sleeping.)

Play is important to infants, to help with learning about their environment. Great care should be taken when choosing toys for infants and government legislation affords some protection for children's toys. Lead-free paint is one example. Toys should be non-toxic and have no detachable or dangerous parts. They should be fireproof, not allow tiny fingers to become trapped nor allow the child to wrap them round part of their body.

Environmental hazards are considered under other headings and in Chapter 8.

The toddler 1–3 years

The toddler years are usually the most difficult for parents, as far as safety is concerned. The toddler is active, inquisitive and extremely mobile, and is often disobedient with little regard for safety.

Provision of a constant temperature

(Refer also to Chapter 5, Maintaining body temperature.)

Toddlers cannot regulate their environment to maintain body temperature. Children in this age group are at risk of febrile convulsions.

Because the pursuit of independence is important to toddlers, they now play outdoors as well as inside and must be correctly dressed to keep warm (see also Chapter 7, Eliminating, personal cleansing and dressing).

Protection from infection

The toddler has started to produce his own antibodies to protect against some infections. The immunisation programme should provide protection against severe diseases.

Provision of a balanced diet and protection from ingesting harmful substances

(Refer also to Chapter 6, Eating and drinking.)

The dangers of incorrectly prepared milk feeds no longer apply to the toddler, but diets must consider foodstuffs which will assist growth and development and protect against infection.

The danger now is ingestion of brightly coloured fluids, tablets and other substances. New experiences are still tested through the mouth, and toddlers are attracted to household fluids kept under the kitchen sink. Cupboards should be kept locked and medicines kept in a childproof cabinet, locked and out of reach. Medicines should also be in childproof containers, although experiments have shown that school children can undo these.

Safety in the kitchen should also be considered. Knives, scissors and other gadgets should be out of reach. Cups of tea and boiling kettles should not be placed near toddlers, who can be accidentally scalded.

Provision of safe playthings

(Refer to Chapter 8, Mobilising, working, playing and sleeping.)

With time toddlers' play becomes more adventurous – riding pedalled vehicles, for example. Often this age group attend clubs and playgroups, where safety must be of prime concern to the supervisors. As toddlers experiment with play toys, by taking them apart, as well as 'toddling' around the house and garden at speed, parents do need 'eyes in the back of the head' to protect their young child from harm.

Environmental hazards

Toddlers can walk up (and tumble down) stairs, so gates or barriers should be fixed at the top and bottom of the stairway. Electrical sockets should be covered and electrical appliances kept out of reach, without the lead dangling, as soon as babies are mobile by rolling or crawling (six months plus).

Windows should be lockable and doors to the outside fitted with proper locks. Doors should not be left ajar, otherwise small fingers can become trapped if the door closes. Chairs and tables should not be put under windows for toddlers to climb on.

Toddlers must be supervised at bath times and with most activities of living.

In the garden, ponds should be covered and play items, such as swings, only used under supervision.

In the car, babies should be restrained from birth, in the back, strapped in a suitable chair and the car should have childproof windows and doors.

The preschool and school child 3–11 years

During the preschool and school years, there is an increased understanding of safety, although experimentation still leads children into dangerous situations. Children of this age begin to learn from and remember accidents and dangerous situations, but they may still forget this at times of distraction or when they are busy playing.

Provision of a constant temperature

(Refer to Chapter 5, Maintaining body temperature.)

Preschool and school children begin to regulate their external environment by putting on and taking off clothes. The likelihood of febrile convulsions diminishes by the school years.

Protection from infection

Increased sociability in the preschool and school years places this age group at greater risk from acquired infections. The immunisation programme will now be complete until adolescence when further immunisation takes place (see Table 2.2). Young children are prone to coughs and colds but usually overcome these without treatment.

Environmental hazards

In the house, preschool and school children are by now more safety-conscious and to aid comprehension, dangers should be explained. School children enjoy increased responsibility in relation to household tasks, but these should be supervised, for instance with cooking. Burns and scalds are still possible from bathwater which is too hot and a child can drown in a few inches of water.

This age group are easily led and distracted by play and other children. Accidents on the road become a real danger and teaching of the Green Cross Code is essential. Care with equipment in the playground such as swings and climbing frames and care during sports should be achieved by the supervision of a teacher. The school has a responsibility to keep play areas safe, for example ensuring that ground surfaces under swings will not cause head or other injuries if the child falls. New, very active play, such as tree climbing and cycle riding, is not without dangers and some minor bumps and grazes are inevitable. Seatbelts should continue to be worn and children should still travel in the rear of the car. A point worth noting is that children of this age who 'babysit' for siblings are not really aware of all the dangers in the home and how to deal, for instance, with fire.

The adolescent 11–18 years

Comprehension of safety should be well developed in the adolescent. However, adolescents often experiment with their worlds in order to discover their own identities. This can be dangerous to health.

Protection from infection

Immunisations in adolescence include the BCG against tuberculosis (if Mantoux-negative) and the rubella vaccine for girls.

Table 2.3 The legal status of the adolescent (Steinberg 1981)

AGE	STATUS
10 years	Child reaches age of criminal responsibility.
12 years	May buy a pet.
14 years	May own an airgun. May be taken into a bar by an adult, but may not be bought an alcoholic drink.
16 years	May buy cigarettes. May consent or withhold consent to medical treatment. Girls may be given contraceptive help without parental involvement.
17 years	May live away from home without parental consent. May be given a prison (or Borstal) sentence.
18 years	Achieves full adult rights including marrying without parental consent. May buy and consume intoxicating drinks in a public house. Has the right to vote. May no longer be taken into care by the local authority.

Alterations in hormonal balance may predispose the adolescent to acne and other minor infections, also changes in diet may alter the immune status.

When beginning sexual relationships, the adolescent may be predisposed to sexually transmitted diseases. This topic is one that should be carefully discussed at school and at home.

Environmental hazards

Environmental hazards to the adolescent range from motorcycle and car accidents to pregnancy and abortion. In the latter case, contraception should be discussed at home and, within legal constraints, be part of the school health education programme.

Some adolescents have already experimented with 'abusive' practices during the school years. These include glue sniffing, drug taking, alcohol consumption and smoking. Patterns established in the school and adolescent years are often difficult to change and the adolescent is often not interested in the long-term consequences of self-inflicted harm.

Health education campaigns are often aimed at this age group, through media, newspapers and journal advertisements. The most effective message may be through an adolescent's role model, which may be the 'right or wrong message'.

Children with special needs

Children who have not developed fully, mentally or physically, will need constant vigilance throughout their lives. They may never develop an awareness of safety (refer to Chapter 8, Guidelines for a care plan for Paul, a schoolchild with cerebral palsy).

Safety in the paediatric ward

The nurse in paediatrics must consider safety of the environment an essential component of planning care for the individual child. Knowledge of the child's safety cognition at differing developmental stages may assist with this.

General safety principles

A children's ward should look homely and bright. There should be provision for play and room for families to visit and be resident. Safety must be aimed at the whole family, while the child is hospitalised.

All children should be easily identifiable by wearing a legible and accurate identification band around their wrist or ankle.

Some unsafe situations in the paediatric ward include wet floors, toys left in corridors and polythene bags within children's reach. Doors should have high handles and windows should be kept locked. Beds, lockers, tables and chairs should all be in correct working order. The nursing staff should know what action to take in the case of a fire or other major accident.

The ward should be kept at a constant temperature, especially the cubicles where infants are nursed.

Children who are admitted with an infection or who are susceptible to infection should be nursed in isolation in a specially equipped cubicle.

Isolation nursing

There are two types of isolation nursing: source isolation and protective isolation.

1 Source isolation

This type of isolation is used to nurse a child who has an infection and to protect other children in the ward from the source of the infection.

Infection may be transmitted by droplet, touch or through blood or elimination products. Nurses, medical, paramedical and ancillary staff may be the vectors, also parents and children may transmit the infection.

Examples include gastroenteritis, meningitis (until organism isolated), hepatitis or HIV-positive children with an open wound or drain.

2 Protective isolation

This type of isolation is used to nurse children who are susceptible to infection and to protect them from infection from other children in the ward. Infection may be transmitted to the child by any of the above named 'source' routes or by any personnel. Infants are particularly susceptible to infection, as are children who are severely ill or immunocompromised as in a leukaemic relapse or where the child has been badly burned.

EXERCISE

Check your local health authority policy on isolation nursing before commencing this exercise.

1 By what routes can infection be spread to other children from the child who is isolated?

Local policy Every health authority has a policy for isolation nursing. This should include differing types of isolation, which diseases should be isolated, and preparation of a cubicle or side room.

Check if your health authority policy further subdivides source isolation into categories to account for the differing routes of transmission of infection.

The cubicle environment should be safe, tidy and homely. Some rooms have their own ventilation systems and others have an *en suite* bathroom. This is particularly useful for the older child in isolation.

2 Using the example of a 3-month-old infant with an excoriated sore bottom and with diarrhoea (of unknown cause) consider the following questions:

Source isolation
The main principle involved in nursing a child in source isolation is to prevent the spread of the infection to others in the ward.

a) When would it be necessary to wash your hands in the care of this infant?
b) How would you dispose of the following items from the source isolation cubicle?
   (i) Burnable rubbish
   (ii) Linen and clothes
   (iii) Nappies, potties and bedpans
   (iv) Feeding equipment and eating utensils
   (v) Play items
   (vi) Medical equipment (e.g. stethoscope, auroscope)
c) How may the room need cleaning during and after the infected child's occupation?

Protective isolation
The principle involved here is to protect the infant or child from infection, because they are particularly at risk.

3 When would it be unwise for you (the student nurse) to care for a child in protective isolation?

The cubicle environment should be safe, homely and tidy, as in source isolation.

4 What factors would you consider before taking any equipment into a protective isolation cubicle?

5 When would it be necessary to wash your hands and how does this differ from source isolation nursing?

Care of the family whose child is isolated

Families are often frightened of caring for their child when in isolation. They need careful and practical explanations of the principles involved. Once parents have been educated, they are often very willing to be included in care and can be an asset to the ward team. Siblings should be able to visit, but preferably kept away from other children in the ward. Parents can get very lonely if they are confined to a cubicle, particularly if they are resident. Any plan of care must incorporate frequent visits to talk with parents and encourage them to take meal breaks.

1 List the points which should be taught to the following personnel likely to enter an isolation cubicle:
   a) parents and relatives;
   b) medical and paramedical staff; and
   c) ancillary staff.

Children's reactions to isolation

Infants appear to accept isolation by sleeping a lot, however they need comfort and stimulation just as they do when they are well.

Toddlers and preschool children do not like being isolated, regarding this enclosure as a restriction of freedom and sometimes as a punishment. Extra nursing time must be spent with this age group in isolation. School children need a lot to do and need to be able to see what is going on outside. Isolation is still not liked, but is better accepted than with young children. Adolescents like privacy and their own room, however when isolation is necessary they should not be left alone for too long as they often need company and reassurance.

Safety in relation to children admitted for operations or investigations under anaesthesia

To illustrate pre- and post-operative safety an Activities of Living framework has been chosen for a four-year-old child admitted for planned surgery.

The admission of children to a paediatric ward, including the principles of taking a nursing history, is discussed more fully in Chapter 3.

Fig. 2.1 Nursing history sheet

NURSING HISTORY SHEET

Date of admission: 2.10.87 **Date of Assessment:** 2.10.87

Surname: Payne **Forenames:** Sophie Jane

Male/Female: F **Age:** 4 years

Date of Birth: 19.7.84 **Nationality:** British

Prefers to be addressed as: Sophie

Address of usual residence: 9 Portside Road, Mumbletown, Portsmouth.

Type of accommodation: Semi-detached house

Family/others at this residence: Mother, father, Steven and Helen

Next of kin: **Name(s):** Mr and Mrs Payne

Relationship: Mother and father

Address: As above

Telephone: Mumbletown 226

Occupation: **Father:** Salesperson

Mother: Housewife, part-time shop assistant

Significant others: (relatives/dependants) As above and maternal grandmother

School: Mumbletown Preschool Group

Religious beliefs and relevant practices: R/C

Patient's perception of current health status: Got to have lump taken away

General practitioner: Mrs Dickie, Mumbletown 535

Reasons for admission/referral: Femoral hernia

Medial diagnosis: As above

Past medical history: Nothing significant

Allergies: None known

Significant life crisis: Starting preschool group

CARE PLAN

A four-year-old girl admitted for femoral hernia repair

Sophie Payne was admitted on the afternoon prior to the day of her operation for correction of femoral hernia. If she had lived nearer the hospital she could have been admitted as a day patient, but this was not practical for the family, as the travelling involved was too great and too expensive.

Sophie's normal routines were assessed using the Activities of Living framework (refer to Chapter 1). The problems, actual and potential, arising from this assessment are shown in a pre-operative care plan (Fig. 2.2). The first three activities of living have been used to structure the care plan.

Fig. 2.2 Pre-operative care plan for Sophie Payne

Problem	Goal and nursing action and rationale	Evaluation
Communicating (A of L) Anxiety about new environment, especially as Sophie has recently been upset with starting the preschool group.	**Goal** Minimise anxiety by explaining all new procedures to Sophie and family. **Nursing action and rationale** Allow time to settle and ask questions and to complete the nursing history. Explain all new procedures using simple language and role play. Mum will need to know all aspects of pre- and post-operative care and how she can assist. Introduce to play therapist and other children. Show around ward, bed and play area. Identify mum's bed and parent sitting room. Give mum meal vouchers. Ensure siblings are involved and not jealous. It is extremely important to explain to children the procedure they will undergo to prevent behaviours associated with stress.	Sophie was given bed number 3, in the open ward with other preschool and school children. She settled slowly, wishing to be close to mum. Sophie joined the children for pre-operative role play, dressing up as a nurse. Dad arrived to collect Steven and Helen in the evening. He was to phone the ward on returning home.

Fig. 2.2 *cont.*

Problem	Goal and nursing action and rationale	Evaluation
Maintaining a safe environment (A of L) (p) New environment and associated safety factors. (p) Hazards associated with an anaesthetic and operation.	**Goal** Prepare Sophie safely for operation and prevent environmental accidents. **Nursing action and rationale** Sophie was identified with a correctly written name band on her wrist. She was weighed, temperature and pulse recordings were taken and a 4-hourly observation chart commenced and her urine tested. Mum ensured she had no hairclips, jewellery or nail varnish on and bathed Sophie the night before operation. The nurse checked her hair for cleanliness and her mouth for loose teeth. Mum also assisted the doctor in the examination Sophie required. The doctor explained the procedure so that Mrs Payne understood the operation. A consent form was then signed and dated. The following morning Sophie was encouraged to pass urine to empty her bladder. Her bed was made up with clean linen. A pre-operative check list may be used to ensure the child is not predisposed to dangers associated with operations (i.e. correct premedication dosage, correct identification, post-operative urinary retention).	Weight: 16.0kg. T: 36.8°C. P: 100 per min. Urine: NAD Sophie had pierced ears and earrings were removed. No infestation noted. Sophie was not very cooperative with the examination. Consent form checked for completion. Small amount of urine passed. Check list completed.
Breathing (A of L) (p) Obstruction of airway pre- and post-operatively.	**Goal** Ensure airway remains patent pre- and post-operatively. **Nursing action and rationale** Give last glucose drink 4–6 hours pre-operatively (consult local policy) then nothing by mouth. This minimises vomiting and airway obstruction. Ensure child has no food hidden in locker or bed. Put a sign on the bed and one pinned to Sophie saying 'I must not eat or drink'. Sophie's premedication was ordered 2 hours pre-operatively; a pleasant-tasting oral medicine. Premedications are given to sedate the child and dry secretions, thus minimising inhalation.	Small amount of fluid taken by 6a.m. Mum has removed all food and drink. Sophie was proud of her badge. Premedication taken with persuasion from mum.

Eventually Sophie fell asleep from the medication. The porter arrived to take her to theatre and the accompanying nurse checked it was the correct child. This pre-operative check should include Sophie's identiband, notes and the treatment card and that she has received pre-medication at the correct time. Mrs Payne was able to accompany Sophie into the anaesthetic room and stay until she was anaesthetised. This is a controversial subject as not all hospitals see the benefit of parents being present during the child's anaesthesia induction or during recovery. Providing parents are well prepared for what to expect, their presence can be very beneficial to the child.

During the time the child is in theatre, parents often appreciate somewhere to sit and a cup of tea or coffee. They will also appreciate regular information about their child.

The nurse should prepare the bed area to receive the child back safely from the recovery room. Oxygen and suction should be available and in correct working order; a vomit bowl and tissues must also be at hand. Charts are needed for recording observations. Special items which the child associates with life outside hospital should be placed within sight of the child's bed.

The immediate post-operative plan of care for Sophie is given in Fig. 2.3. The first three activities of living have been used for the immediate period, as these are most applicable to the child after anaesthetic and operation. By using only three, the plan may become more realistic in a busy paediatric ward. Subsequent care should consider *all* activities of living.

The plan outlines only the immediate post-operative care necessary to maintain a safe environment for the child. Subsequent care, dependent on the child's recovery and length of stay in hospital, would necessitate consideration of all problems arising from the 12 Activities of Living.

Fig. 2.3 Post-operative care plan (immediate) for Sophie Payne, following surgery for a femoral hernia

Problem	Goal and nursing action and rationale	Evaluation
Breathing (A of L) (p) Airway obstruction due to altered conscious level following anaesthesia, and/or due to (p) Vomiting	**Goal** Maintain a clear airway until consciousness fully regained. **Nursing action and rationale** Position Sophie in the Recovery position. Observe level of consciousness and general colour. Commence ½-hourly observations of pulse and respirations and 4-hourly temperature. Withhold fluids until fully conscious. Clean mouth with soft swabs.	Sophie was semi-conscious on returning to the ward with mum. Her colour was pale, but not cyanosed. P: 110 per min. R: 24 per min. She was too sleepy to ask for fluids. No vomiting in the first 3 hours post-operatively.
(p) Bleeding from abdominal wound site.	Observe wound ½-hourly. Mark on dressing any bleeding which has occurred. Reassure Sophie and mum if concerned. Minimise mobilisation and touching wound site.	Small amount of blood on dressing, no marking as minimal dressing over wound site and wound visible underneath.
Communicating (A of L) Pain at wound site.	**Goal** Prevent pain. **Nursing action and rationale** Observe Sophie carefully for pain (i.e. crying, restlessness, pale colour, holding stomach). Give prescribed analgesia if pain observed. Check effect at ½-hour and 2 hours later. Note if Sophie sleeps.	Analgesia given on return to the ward, as Sophie was crying and saying it hurt. Effect after ½-hour - drowsiness and no complaints of pain.
Anxiety following operation (and associated with pain).	Ensure mum understands the operation so she can assist in the explanation to Sophie. Familiar objects such as toys, cuddlies and photos should be nearby the child. Ensure child feels she has not been punished and reassure her that she will get better. Touch and non-verbal communication are very important and help allay anxiety.	Sophie wanted her mother to hold her hand and be with her. She also clutched a hanky of her mother's.
Maintaining a safe environment (A of L) Inability to maintain a safe environment due to effect of anaesthetic, wound site and strange environment.	**Goal** Promote a safe environment. **Nursing action and rationale** Sophie to be kept on bedrest, lying flat until fully conscious. If mum leaves the cot, then the sides must be placed upright. All medicines must be given according to health authority policy.	A safe environment was maintained.
(p) Infection at wound site.	**Goal** Early detection of a wound infection.	

Fig. 2.3 *cont.*

Problem	Goal and nursing action and rationale	Evaluation
	Nursing action and rationale Infection is not likely to be observed until 24 or more hours later. However, monitoring the child immediately post-operatively may ensure early detection of infection. 4-hourly temperature recordings should be commenced.	T at 2p.m.: 36.6°C. T at 6p.m.: 36.8°C.
(p) Urinary retention due to anaesthesia and position of wound site.	**Goal** Prevent urinary retention and discomfort.	
	Nursing action and rationale Ensure urine is passed within 12 hours of anaesthesia. Offer a bedpan or carry to toilet. Ensure privacy and cleanliness maintained.	Urine passed 6 hours after operation.

Discharge from hospital

This topic is discussed more fully in Chapter 3. However, it is worth noting that parents should feel able to care for their child on discharge and to receive a written set of guidelines for the child's aftercare. This supports the concept of safe care following surgery.

Administration of medicines

Care must be taken when administering medicines to any age group. Children are unaware of the dangers of medicines and extra precautions must be taken, for example checking their identiband. Painful injections are avoided whenever possible.

Local policy

Every health authority has a policy for Administration of Medicines. This should include who may administer and how and when to administer medicines. Guidelines should also be included on the importance of weighing children and the calculation of medicines.

Calculation of medicines

A simple calculation should be used.

$$\frac{\text{Amount prescribed}}{\text{Amount on stock bottle or ampoule.}} \times \frac{\text{Dilution on stock bottle or ampoule}}{1}$$

or

$$\frac{\text{What you want}}{\text{What you've got}} \times \frac{\text{Amount of dilution}}{1}$$

e.g. Ampicillin 125 mg prescribed. Stock bottle 250 mg in 5 ml.

Therefore $\frac{125\text{ mg}}{250\text{ mg}} \times \frac{5\text{ ml}}{1}$

$$\frac{125}{250} \times \frac{5}{1} = \frac{1}{2} \times \frac{5}{1} = \frac{5}{2} = 2.5\text{ ml}$$

EXERCISE

Test your calculations for the following medicines:

1 The child is prescribed Atropine 0.4 mg orally and the stock bottle contains 0.6 mg in 5 ml.
Calculate the amount the child requires.

2 The child is prescribed Digoxin 0.02 mg orally and the stock bottle holds 0.05 mg in 1 ml.
Calculate the amount the child requires.

3 The child is prescribed an injection of 32 mg of a medicine and the stock ampoule is 80 mg in 1 ml.
Calculate the amount required.

Answers

1 $\frac{0.4}{0.6} \times \frac{5}{1} = \frac{4}{6} \times \frac{5}{1} = \frac{10}{3} = 3.33\text{ ml}$

2 $\frac{0.02}{0.05} \times \frac{1}{1} = \frac{2}{5} \times \frac{1}{1} = \frac{2}{5} = 0.4\text{ ml}$

3 $\frac{32}{80} \times \frac{1}{1} = \frac{4}{10} = 0.4\text{ ml}$

Caring for blood transfusions and intravenous infusions

(Refer also to Chapter 4, Care Plan for Florence Mercury in sickle cell crisis and to Chapter 6, Eating and drinking, care of an intravenous infusion.)

Transfusions or infusions set up on children must be very carefully regulated to the rate prescribed by the doctor. Reactions to blood products are likely to occur sooner and more severely than in adults. For instance, if a child reacts to blood products with a pyrexia, it could lead to a febrile convulsion. Overloading the child's system with fluid causing oedema could precipitate breathlessness and cyanosis.

Apart from the physiological effects of transfusions and infusions, from a practical stance, children can become entangled in the tubing, and it is possible they can strangle themselves. As the cannula and tubing are restrictive to movement, children try to remove them and have been known to cut the tubing with scissors!

Preparation of milk feeds and infant feeding

Refer to Chapter 6, Eating and drinking for guidance on preparation and calculation of feeds and infant feeding.

Observations – physical and psychological

Never be frightened to report an observational change if you are unsure of the consequences. Better to be safe than sorry.

Observing children for changes in activities of living and the problems associated with this are considered in the following chapters. However, it is worth mentioning that the slightest change in a child you are observing is worth reporting. Listen to what parents tell you; very often if they think their child is better or worse, they are right.

Provision of safe toys

Refer to Chapter 8, Mobilising, working, playing and sleeping for safety aspects concerning toys.

Child abuse

Child abuse is considered in this chapter because if a child is abused, there has been a failure of safe care for the child.

This is a sensitive and emotive topic and often promotes strong reactions from nursing and medical staff. The nurse caring for a child who is admitted with suspected child abuse should not be judgemental in her attitude to the parents, although this is not always an easy situation. The background factors which have led to this failure of care may have been immense for the parents. Very often they feel guilty, upset and frightened of the consequences of their actions. In other cases, the parent(s) need to be prosecuted for their action and these situations are often taken up by the media.

Children in the paediatric ward who are admitted with suspected abuse are often waiting for a case conference to decide their future. A Place of Safety Order may have been secured from a Magistrate to hold the child for 28 days to sort out the family situation.

The nurses' role at this time is to observe the relationship between the family and the child and to do this is a sensitive and caring manner.

Further consideration of abuse, that of sexual abuse, will be considered in Chapter 9, Expressing sexuality.

REFERENCES

DHSS. 1984. *Immunisation against infectious diseases*, prepared by the Joint Committee on Vaccination and Immunisation for the Secretary of State for Social Services. DHSS, London.

DEPARTMENT OF TRADE AND INDUSTRY. 1987. *Home Accident Surveillance System*, 10th Annual Report 1986 Data. Chairman Hon Francis Maude MP, Department of Trade and Industry (Consumer Safety Unit).

HANSON, L. 1987. No Longer the Nit Lady. *Nursing Times*, **83**(22), 30–32.

MOON, A. 1987. Pictures of Health. ABPN Spotlight on Children in *Nursing Times*, **83**(1), 49–50.

STEINBERG, D. 1981. Normal Development in Adolescence. *Midwife, Health Visitor and Community Nurse*, **17**(11).

UNITED KINGDOM CENTRAL COUNCIL 1986. *Administration of Medicines: A UKCC Advisory Paper*. A framework to assist individual professional judgement and the development of local policies and guidelines. UKCC, London.

FURTHER READING

DHSS. 1984. *AIDS Interim Guidelines*. Advisory Committee on Dangerous Pathogens (revised June 1986). HMSO, London.

OFFICE OF POPULATION, CENSUSES, AND SURVEYS. 1986. *Mortality Statistics 1984*. HMSO, London.

3 Communicating

Effective communication is a basic principle of all nursing care and in paediatrics its importance cannot be overemphasised. The nurse must be prepared to spend time explaining to children all new and especially frightening experiences, so that the child maintains trust in his caregivers. As paediatric care involves the whole family, it is important that parents in particular are included in discussions about care and treatment and they need explanations so that their worries are minimised. The freedom of working with and communicating with parents must be balanced by the need for confidentiality.

Consideration is given in this chapter to pain and stress in children. To identify pain in infants and small children, the nurse needs to use all her observational skills, as non-verbal communication may be the only way in which a young child can express pain. Likewise, stress and anxiety in children may not be shown verbally, but by small non-verbal clues.

How children communicate

Non-verbal communication

Children communicate many feelings through non-verbal expression. This may include facial changes, body posture and language and the child's general manner and attitude. A frightened child may resort to earlier (regressive) behaviour, may become shy and clinging or alternatively may become very noisy and naughty.

Children often use toys to express how they feel, performing on the toy what in turn has happened to them (e.g. hitting or shaking a doll). This use of toys is currently being employed by those working with children to determine whether sexual abuse has occurred (see Chapter 9).

Verbal communication

Consideration is given below to how children communicate at differing developmental stages. It is important to note that crying, temper tantrums and laughter are all forms of verbal communication and may be useful to note in children who cannot speak.

Infant communication

Infants make their wishes known by crying or movement. Usually cries represent an unpleasant stimulus such as a wet or soiled nappy or hunger.

At first faces which appear in front of the infant are black, grey or white, and blurred at the edges. Cones in the retina of the eye (for colour perception) begin to mature after birth and slowly the infant perceives colours and accommodation associated with clear vision. The infant is attracted by the eyes and mouth of the face nearby. At first the infant centres on observing these aspects, and this highlights the importance of the carer's non-verbal communication. The infant can hear and makes little noises, 'jumping' if suddenly moved or if there is a loud noise. Touch is very important and the infant likes to be held firmly and securely, while being cuddled and spoken to softly.

Accommodation is the movement of the muscles of the eye which enable the lens to become more convex to focus, especially for near vision.

By eight weeks of age eye coordination is advanced so that light and objects are looked at. Sounds made nearby make the infant stop to listen. The infant coos, squeals and starts to smile, so that by 12 weeks a full social smile is seen. Babbling emerges, as does familiarity with faces and objects which are recognised.

At 16 weeks, the infant turns the head to a familiar sound and can recognise mum, laughing and chuckling and engaging in reciprocal 'chat' with parents if eye-to-eye contact is maintained.

In the second half of the first year, the infant recognises the family and therefore begins to identify and become wary of strangers. Primitive words emerge such as 'da-da' and 'ba-ba'. The more encouragement that is received the more the infant will try to talk. The direction of sound is clearly localised by the eighth month and it is possible for the health visitor or GP to test for hearing perception (to loud and soft sounds). At ten months, the infant responds to its own name, makes facial expressions and sounds and looks at picture books.

At the end of the first year, a preference for one or other hand will be seen, as will the ability to indicate wants and needs by pointing. Two or three specific words are verbalised and many infants enjoy music.

Toddlers' and preschool children's communication

By toddler age, the development of language is dramatic, for instance at 18 months, ten words are discernible whereas by two years, 200–300 words are spoken. Phrases are used at first, which develop into short sentences. Imitation, which furthers the toddler's learning, can be very tiring and irritating. Repeating words heard ('echolalia') is evident at this age. Simple commands are obeyed, but there is no understanding of right or wrong.

Transitional objects, often given by parents as comforters, are important and must not be mislaid. These may be play items or pieces of blanket, nightdresses or hankies. They represent the parent and 'stand in' for them when they are not with the toddlers. Although toddlers understand better than infants that when a parent is out of sight they will return, they still do not tolerate this well.

Communication and thought are egocentric, so that everything focuses on 'me', the child, 'how will *I* feel'. This continues up to school age. Children of this age use mobility and touch if they want to change a situation, so that a toy they want will be pulled towards them, whereas strangers will be pushed away. Pointing is also a means of saying what is wanted.

By three years of age, the vocabulary comprises 900 words and among the most commonly used are 'why?', 'what?', and 'when?'. Communication and play still revolve around the individual child but some indications are noted that the child may begin to consider sharing. 'No' is the word used a lot of the time, even if the reverse is meant. Children stamp their independence on life and 'no' is one representation of this. Likewise, temper tantrums may arise from the child's frustration at not being able to do something, either because of physical inability or because parents have not allowed it.

Gender roles are identified, but boys and girls may still respond to each other without making sexual distinctions.

At four years, language has progressed to include aggression and profanities and simple explanations are required about cause and effect. Around 1500 words are recognisable and incessant questioning continues. The child knows the colours and can draw shapes which are recognisable, but without detail. When colouring drawings the child does not keep within the lines.

By school time, communication in the verbal, written and expressive fields should have equipped the child to learn new information and to work and play with other children. For instance, the child has a vocabulary of 2100 words and talks constantly, enjoying participating in conversations. Most children at five years can print their first name and other simple words, can name their address, state their age, count to ten and name the days of the week.

It is possible to talk about 'tomorrow', as the child begins to think in terms of time units, but usually requires 'staging points' along the way (i.e. 'one dinner and one sleep before tomorrow').

Imagination has played a key part through the preschool years. Imaginary friends and 'magical thinking' are processes through which the child may pass. Children often talk to inanimate objects, or to people and friends who are not in sight and, particularly in play, use their imagination. This may also extend to fears formed in their mind or associated with characters seen in books or on the television. Children also have consciences and understand when they have 'done wrong', but the difference between right and wrong only emerges when the child reaches school age.

School children's communication

The young school child continues to print and draw, at first using large letters, which do not always stay on the ruled line. The drawings are representative of thoughts and the child also begins to read. By the age of eight, script writing in sentences is seen. The child thinks more about life and what is learnt and likes logical conclusions and endings. Monetary value is learned.

In the older school years (i.e. 9–11 years) there is good hand–eye coordination and this is applied in writing, drawing, sports, hobbies and general mobility. Any activities undertaken can be broken into steps, with the child being able to plan in advance. Learning is enjoyed, memory develops and work at school becomes competitive. The self-centredness of the young child is lost during early school years and sharing both in play and life in general is seen. The older school children can plan to visit places and do so on their own. However, safety must be maintained and many parents like to accompany their children on visits and excursions.

Adolescent communication

Adolescents can discuss and debate subjects, beginning to think conceptually and to be aware of past, present and future. Knowledge is acquired at a rapid speed and this is utilised in school work and life generally. Adolescents develop a language and a culture of their own, with special words known only to themselves and their friends. There is often a reticence to talk with parents, a moodiness if forced to participate in family outings, whereas with their peer group, adolescents can be talkative and noisy. Much language and behaviour is modelled on idols and heroes and influenced by television programmes. By this age, the adolescent is working out his position in life, often brooding about and idealising over his future life and this can be reflected in his communication.

Cognitive and psychosocial development which affect communication

Development of cognitive thought

Piaget (1969) spent considerable time establishing the stages through which children's cognition develops. He suggested the following stages:

1 *Sensori-motor 0–2 years*
The child assimilates and accommodates information from his world by sight, hearing, touch and movement. Everything which he touches he draws towards him in a circular movement of his arms. Usually objects are 'tasted' through the mouth. His physical movements reflect the egocentric nature of thought and the child cannot distinguish himself from his mother and father.

2 *Pre-operational 2–7 years*
The term **pre-operation**, means the child cannot conceptualise (**operation** being thinking through actions in the mind). He remains egocentric at the beginning of this phase, using 'I', 'Me', 'I want' language. Any reasoning fixes on one dimension, for example a short fat glass half full of water is seen to hold less than a tall thin glass filled to the top; but actually contains the same amount of water. (This was one of Piaget's experiments with children.) In another sphere, because the man in the child's family is usually his daddy, then all men must be daddies. This type of thought is called **transductive reasoning**. Pre-operational children also give life and intention to inanimate objects, so that if they run into a table and hurt themselves, they tell the table off and often smack it as well. This is known as **animism**. One other related point about this age group, is that thought is very literal. For example, Pontious (1981) described how the term 'hold your horses' was used to tell a child to 'wait a minute'. The child went to find some toy horses to hold and asked if the time was right now? Literal also includes thinking in black and white, so that if a pain hurts, it hurts, *not* a little or a lot. It either hurts or it doesn't.

3 *Concrete operations 7–11 years*
By this stage, the child has a more realistic view of the world and will accept that other people have views too. Egocentricity disappears as the child has a good understanding of his own body boundaries and personal identity. He can see both sides of a situation, this being called **reversibility**. It is also possible for the child to identify degrees, for instance of time, day, size and mass. A pain in the body will now be a lot or a little, in other words, less black and white than in the preoperational stage. The child's thinking is realistic, but he still cannot hypothesise, as yet being unable to form mental images (concepts).

4 *Formal operations 11 years onwards*
The final Piagetan stage completes the development of thought. The adolescent can form mental pictures and can carry out activities in the mind (operations). He can hypothesise and use abstract thought.

Table 3.1 Five stages of psychosocial development in children, according to Erikson and Freud (from Lewer & Robertson, 1987)

ERIKSON	AGE	FREUD
1 Sense of trust	0–1 years	Oral stage
Mothering important – relationship with one person.		
2 Sense of autonomy	1–3 years	Anal stage
Autonomy symbolised by the holding or letting go of the sphincter muscles. Increasing ability to control themselves and their bodies and environment.		
3 Sense of initiative	3–6 years	Genital/phallic
Strong imagination. Conscience develops. Guilt develops. Freud says Oedipal phase – child forms an attachment to parent of opposite sex.		
4 Sense of industry	6–12 years	Latency
Ready to be workers and producers. Want to carry tasks through to completion.		
5 Sense of identity	12–18 years	Puberty
Rapid physical change. Over-occupied with appearance in sight of others.		

Psychosocial development

Piaget's work was mainly concerned with cognitive development. However, Freud and Erikson wrote extensively on the psychological and social development of the child. Freud in particular has received criticism of the stages he suggested of psychological development. Much of his work can be noted in children, such as the desire to 'hold on' or 'let go' in the toddler years (anal stage). A comparison of some of the key points from the work of Freud and Erikson is given in Table 3.1.

Communicating with the family

In the community

In order to bring up a child and enhance his development, parents bear a responsibility for communicating with and teaching their child. In some families this is helped by grandparents and other relatives who may live nearby, thus forming an extended family network. Advice on child rearing is often sought from those who have already undergone the experience, such as grandmothers and neighbours. The influence of such family members and friends may be the most acceptable to new parents.

Help and advice from professionals are available both before and after the birth of the infant, the midwife being responsible for mum and baby until the tenth day, then the health visitor looking after the child until five years. The health visitor or the general practitioner will developmentally assess the child at around 6 weeks, 7 and 15 months and 2½ years, the assessment including hearing tests (after 7–8 months) and assessment of verbal skills. When the child goes to school, the medical team assess the child annually and the school teacher also has a responsibility for noting the child's verbal and written ability to communicate. If necessary, children are referred to a specialist. Children with speech difficulties can attend speech therapy classes. Deaf children need early home tuition, hearing aids fitted if appropriate (i.e. for those with partial hearing) and decisions made about schooling. Many partially deaf children can attend normal schools, but must sit at the front of the class.

Children who have behaviour problems which can manifest in delayed or inappropriate communication may be helped by a clinical psychologist.

Defects and abnormalities to speech and hearing may require the advice of an ENT paediatric specialist.

Different cultural groups

Britain is a multiracial society and health workers must be prepared to communicate with many cultural groups. Although many activities of living are affected by culture, communication is likely to be the most important. In some areas, health workers who speak languages such as Bengali, Urdu, etc. have been employed to promote health amongst the community. Health education material is also printed in different languages. Communication with these groups will be enhanced if an understanding of the cultural background of the community is known, for instance Indian women may not go out unless escorted, usually by their husbands. Maternal grandmothers may be very influential on the child's upbringing, giving contradictory advice to that of the health workers, for example in the field of medicines.

In hospital

When a child is admitted to hospital (Accident & Emergency, Outpatients Department,

Paediatric Ward), the parents are often as anxious as their offspring. Any communication must include parents and siblings and explanations should be in lay terms with time for discussion and clarification afterwards. Parents can be an asset in outpatients departments and in casualty, whilst also being essential for the sick child in the paediatric ward. Adopt a friendly and informative approach to families, be honest, but maintain confidentiality. Where siblings are involved, to avoid jealousy give them a personal explanation about treatment and care and enlist their help in some small, safe way. Find out what they interpret is happening to their brother or sister and dispel misconceptions.

Resident parents and free visiting

Parents should be made to feel welcome to the ward and areas provided for them to be resident with their child. A kitchen and sitting area are also necessary, as well as free or subsidised meals in the hospital canteen.

If parents cannot be resident, they should not be condemned, but consideration and support given to the whole family situation. Free visiting was established as necessary as long ago as 1959 (Ministry of Health) and supported by the work of Robertson (1953) at The Tavistock Institute. However, some paediatric wards still restrict visiting after operations such as tonsillectomies. Most parents, provided they are given clear explanations, are willing and able to be present during (or following) the most traumatic treatment.

The ward team

Communication between the paediatric ward team members must be accurate and clear for the safety of the child. Where observations are concerned, for instance an infant whose vital signs suddenly alter, or whose colour deteriorates, the need to tell the trained nurse or medical staff immediately may be the difference between life or death. This sounds dramatic, but a young sick child's state may alter rapidly.

The paediatric team consists of may personnel (see Fig. 3.1) and communication must be just as effective between these different disciplines as it should be with the parents and children.

CHECK LIST

Factors to consider when communicating with children

The environment

A friendly, homely atmosphere should welcome a child to hospital, with a play area and toys available. The ward should be warm and children up and about and in their own clothes if well enough. A certain amount of noise should be expected. Areas should be set aside for parents to be resident, to eat and drink and sit and relax.

Safety must be maintained, so ward doors may have high handles, windows should be secured and all equipment safe.

Verbal and non-verbal communications

1 Speak to the child at eye level; that means bending down and not towering over him.
2 Use simple, recognisable language.
3 Use short sentences. Uncomplicated simple phrases and sentences are best for the young child.
4 Use positive language, i.e.: 'Come with Mummy, and we will . . .', not 'Would you like to . . . ?' A young child is not in a position to make such choices and will inevitably say no.
5 Don't scold, or tell children off. This is likely to encourage bad behaviour, or discourage a child from attempting something the next time (for example, using the potty without accidents).
6 Allow the child time to establish a relationship, which will become evident when he starts to initiate conversation with you, or to respond more readily. Children are wary of strangers and therefore cannot be expected to communicate at first.

   Sometimes noisy conversation is also a way of expressing concern, and it should not be considered

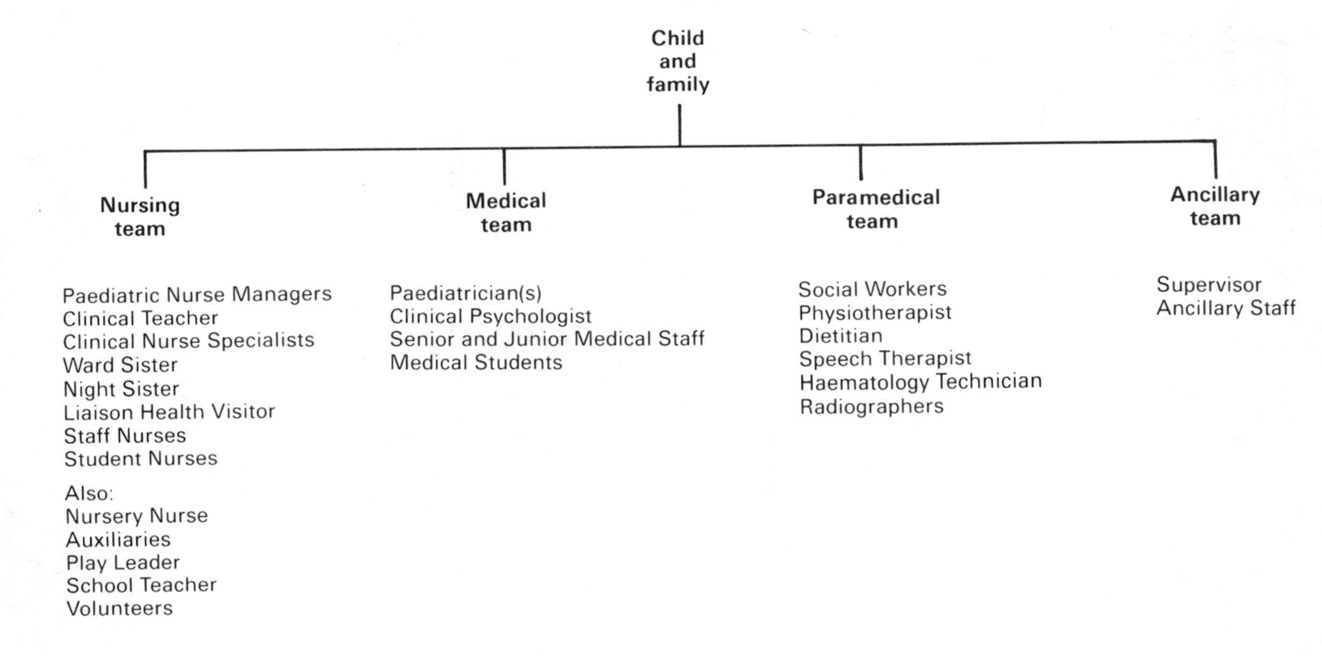

Fig. 3.1 Teams involved with care of the child in the Paediatric Ward

that the child is necessarily either naughty or relaxed and settled.

7 Use touch as a means of communicating. Children respond to gentle and secure handling, to being cuddled and put on laps. Stroking faces and hair may be comforting, as well as showing love and affection to toys. An adolescent may be comforted by a hand on the arm or on the shoulder.
8 Communicate through the child's toys, so that if teddy thinks a medicine tastes nice, then the chances are the child will also like it. Use play also for dressing up in roles (see pre-operative preparation p. 30) and drawings to express feelings.
9 Watch your own non-verbal expressions. Frowns and smiles are noticed by children, as well as attitudes which convey anger, sorrow and happiness. Don't say one thing and let the expression on your face say the other!
10 Above all – be honest!

Preparing children for hospital

Children should be aware of hospitals and their purpose, as part of the everyday life of the community. This is especially important because 45% of children under the age of seven years will have been hospitalised (Davie *et al.* 1972). Children can be introduced to hospital life from an early age, through picture books, toys and television programmes, or may have first-hand experience through visiting siblings in the Special Care or Intensive Care Baby Unit or the paediatric ward.

Children's books may include hospital information in a general way, or may be more specific, such as *Going to the Doctor*, *Visiting the Dentist* or *Going into Hospital*. The National Association for the Welfare of Children in Hospital (NAWCH) produces a wide selection of books and booklets for children of all ages, as well as informing parents about visiting, residency and so on. Playing with dolls is another introduction to hospital and later when the child is older, dressing up and role playing (nurses and doctors) can form part of the learning process. Health visitors play a key role in advising about hospital visits and may provide relevant literature. School teachers can encourage children to write and draw for contemporaries who are hospitalised.

Should children need investigation or examination by a specialist, they usually visit an outpatient department clinic (OPD). Such departments can be made bright, homely and informative and many hospitals employ a play leader to be with the children.

Pre-admission

For children who are visiting the OPD prior to planned surgery, a pre-admission programme can be commenced. As clinics tend to be during the working day (weekdays) some paediatric departments run pre-admission programmes on a Saturday. The programme may include a talk, with a slide or video show about the hospital and having an operation. Children are invited to dress up and play with equipment (masks, stethoscopes, etc.) while parents can ask questions of the nurse and play leader. The visit may also include a short tour of the hospital, including the anaesthetic/recovery room and the paediatric ward, as well as any other relevant departments. Children are given an honest description of what to expect, explained within their limits of understanding. Parents can see what will happen to their child and can give specific answers when at home. School children benefit most from such a programme. Adolescents may like to read relevant literature, use the telephone to ask questions of ward staff or they may like to visit the ward prior to admission. Children of all ages can be encouraged to draw and write about their feelings of being ill or having an operation.

Despite the fact that children admitted to hospital for emergency treatment have not had this preparation time, if they have some knowledge of hospital life, it may help them to be less frightened.

At the basis of all explanation must be openness and honesty, so that children do not lose trust in their parents and, in hospital, in nursing and medical staff. If parents know what to expect, then horror stories can be minimised and hospital not used as a threat.

Admitting and taking a nursing history and making an assessment of the child

When a child is admitted to hospital, first impressions really matter. Follow the check list on page 50 when meeting a child and his family. Admission procedures usually involve observations as well as a ward tour and obtaining information. For most children it is best to let them establish themselves around their beds and locker area and to explore the play room, before attempting to do other aspects of the admission. Unpleasant procedures (such as venepuncture) should be left until the child is settled. Rodin (1983), in her research into preparation given to children before venepuncture, concluded that children (and parents) who are prepared for the procedure are less anxious. In a review of the literature which precedes the research discussion, Rodin notes the contribution of other works such as Hawthorn (1974) which clearly demonstrate the need for parental participation in care to relieve a child's anxiety. Parents and children should not be separated at this time and the child may like to 'hang on' to a favourite toy or cuddly.

When taking a nursing history, attempt to find a quiet, private part of the ward – this can be very difficult in a paediatric ward! Sitting with parents next to the child's bed allows the child to unpack his possessions and establish his own territory. However, remember all information is confidential and not for the ears of every family sitting in the ward!

The nursing history sheet may follow the framework of the Activities of Living (Roper *et al.* 1985) or your paediatric unit may have its own framework. Don't 'fire' questions at parents; they are often frightened and uncertain themselves. Make the process more of a conversation, but write down key points as information is given. Be sensitive to various issues such as potty training which can be a particularly private area for some parents; for example, 'My child is not potty trained. I do not want this to be started in hospital'.

If the 12 Activities of Living are used to form a basis of the child's normal routine, then all areas should be included. Remember that each activity encompasses physical, psychological, socio-cultural, environmental and politico-economic aspects. It might be worth noting that spiritual needs should also be considered.

The most effective way to gain information is to use open-ended questions which let parents explain about their child. Don't forget also, that preschool, school children and adolescents can answer questions for themselves and questions should be directed primarily at the child so that he can attempt to answer.

Parents should be able to read what has been written about their child and can often assist with establishing the problems the child has, or may present (i.e. potential problems).

Once information has been gathered and the child settled, then the family can be shown around the ward. This should include the bathroom and toilet areas and any other places the child may need to use on his own (or under supervision). Observations of temperature, pulse, respirations and blood pressure may form a baseline record, for future changes. Remember that young children don't like things 'taken' from them, so it's better to say 'I'm going to see how warm you are', rather than 'I'm going to *take* your temperature'. Urinalysis may need to be performed when the child feels relaxed enough to urinate. Height and weight are measured for growth and development charts and the weight is needed for medications.

Preparing children for an investigation, treatment or surgery

Explanations to children must be compatible with their stage of development and understanding.

Toddlers cannot usually be prepared for future events until the actual day. They do not comprehend the future and therefore explanations should be simple, short and given just before a procedure. Favourite dolls or toys can be used, for instance to help with a premedication. Parents should really try to be present to explain to toddlers. Cuddles and comfort are needed following a painful experience.

Preschool children can be prepared a little earlier than toddlers, but must have measurable points on which to base a future happening. Young school children also require this sort of staging. Dolls and other toys can be dressed and fitted up for a new experience, such as inserting an infusion, dressing a wound or having ECG leads connected. A child who is about to undergo a similar experience may play with these toys, taking them apart and examining the equipment. An honest explanation of 'how things work' is also necessary. For other children of pre- and school age, books such as *Wiggly's Story* (Foulger 1985) explain about intravenous infusions or there are books with photographs prepared by the ward team, which may show children having a venepuncture or going for surgery.

Children can dress up and act out what they think is going to take place. A play leader and/or a nurse should be available at all times to put right any misconceptions, for example 'they rip your tonsils out'. Adolescents need quiet explanations and seek considerable information in order to understand. Because an adolescent may not ask, it does not mean that he understands; he may be too shy or think he should know, so that he doesn't ask. TV programmes such as the many hospital series can be useful for discussion. As with older school children, adolescents should be prepared well in advance whenever possible. At this age, future happenings are beginning to be conceptualised.

Of course, all this preparation cannot be done where emergency treatment or surgery is necessary. For children in this situation, try to involve the parents, give simple honest explanations to the children and relieve the child's discomfort. The ward photograph book and dolls or toys may be the most suitable aids at such a time. However, often there is no time and explanations must be retrospective once the child has recovered. It is necessary to reflect with the child over what has happened, otherwise when the child returns home he may have reactionary behaviour to the stressful period.

Parents require an explanation and need to give their consent for some investigations and for all treatment under anaesthesia. The consent form is signed by the parent or legal guardian until the child is 16 years old. It is the medical staff's responsibility to explain clearly the treatment to parents, but often it is the nursing staff who follow up this explanation with further details.

The anaesthetic and recovery areas

In some areas it is slowly becoming more acceptable for parents to accompany their child to the anaesthetic room and to be present when the child recovers from anaesthesia. However, not all anaesthetists see the benefit of having parents present during induction, and sometimes theatre nursing staff do not like having parents in the theatre suite. NAWCH continues to campaign on this subject and offers advice and guidance to parents.

If parents are too frightened and do not wish to go with their child to theatre, then a nurse and/or a friend can go with the child. Explanations to parents must be given in advance about wearing a gown, equipment in the anaesthetic room and how their child will be anaesthetised. Likewise, they should know what to expect of their child post anaesthesia, such as a pale facial colour, pain and vomiting.

Where children are accompanied by parents to the theatre suite, premedication may not be necessary. They can wear their own cotton nightclothes and travel in a specially decorated theatre trolley (Fradd 1987).

Parents are advised to leave the room once anaesthesia has made the child unconscious. Often parents need support after this and the nurse can accompany them to the ward or waiting area.

Most recovery area staff like the child to have roused from his unconscious state before parents can be brought to the bedside. The first person any child wants is his mum or dad and having parents available can minimise stress, pain, bleeding and vomiting. Remember parents can be very frightened and upset by other children they see recovering from operation.

Post-operative care

At first, communication with a child following surgery will be through touch and the occasional softly spoken word. It is best to let the child sleep off the anaesthetic, and discourage parents from attempting to rouse him. Let parents see what the child has had done and explain in lay terms what this means. You will need to be prepared to return at a later time to explain further. Parents can stroke faces and hair, hold hands with their child, or when the child will not settle, cuddle him on their lap. Touching or investigating the surgical area should be discouraged. Once the child begins to waken, sips of water and washing hands and face can be done by parents. Pain relief which is very important after procedures must be given regularly and to an adequate level (see p. 64).

Young children can be bewildered by equipment attached to them and once again the nurse must take time to explain, using dolls and toys where appropriate. Preschool children think that their 'insides can leak out' if their skin has been cut or punctured and therefore need reassurance. If the child has had a particularly difficult or painful operation, psychologically it may take him some time to get over this, although his body may heal quickly. Once a child feels better, he usually shows it by activity. A child lying quietly on his bed is not normal!

Going home

Because of the short lengths of stay for children in the paediatric ward, parents need education and support to cope with the child at home. So often advice and teaching are left to the last minute, whereas they should be included from the beginning of care planning. Let parents ask questions and demonstrate care to them, to ensure they understand. It is a good idea for a parent to be performing a skill they will need to do to the child at home, while still in hospital. Besides verbal teaching, parents should have a written set of guidelines to follow. For instance with wound care, parents need to know about preventing infection of the wound, controlling pain and removal of sutures – when and by whom? Also what the child can eat, what he can actively do and therefore play with, can he return to school? and so on.

Sadly, often the only education given is the outpatients appointment date, a letter to the GP and the ward telephone number. Once the child is at home, parents should restablish contact with the health visitor and GP. If specialist help is needed then a paediatric community nurse and/or clinical nurse specialist should have been contacted by the paediatric ward staff.

Many societies and self-help groups can also be useful to the family. (See Societies and useful addresses, p. 181.)

Stress in children

Children become stressed when something occurs which is a change from the usual routine and because of their limited experience, they have difficulty coping.

Stress and anxiety have been important concepts considered throughout the chapter on communication and are a component of many subsequent chapters. Nursing care is aimed at minimising anxiety in children, parents and siblings.

However, it may be useful to know what causes stress at the different developmental stages of childhood and how the child may show this.

Effects of hospitalisation

The main area for concern when young children are hospitalised is to prevent separation

Table 3.2 Stress at different developmental stages

DEVELOPMENTAL STAGE	ANXIETIES	POSSIBLE REACTIONS
1 Infants: trust *v.* mistrust	(i) Bonding – this is part of the maternal child attachment process and behaviour.	Cries Screams Withdraws Resigns himself to situation
	(ii) Sensory motor deprivation or overload, e.g. visual, auditory.	As above
	(ii) Separation from care-giver (after one month and up to eight months).	As above
	(iv) Stranger anxiety from four months.	As above
	(v) Pain.	Cries Has a total body reaction Immobility
2 Toddlers: autonomy *v.* shame and doubt	(i) Separation, as the toddler has an intense mum relationship. (ii) Change in routine and ritual. (iii) Unable to communicate effectively, which increases anxiety. (iv) Loss of autonomy/independence. (v) Loss of body integrity, especially loss of mobility, loss of control and intrusive behaviour. (vi) Pain.	Cries for mum Stops communicating Loses new skills Aggression Tantrums Protest behaviour (see Fig. 3.2)
3 Preschool children: initiative *v.* guilt	(i) Separation – some coping mechanisms, but can't yet cope with separation. (ii) Unfamiliar environments. (iii) Abandonment or punishment (thought of, as loss of parental love). (iv) Body image and integrity (mutilation, loss of identity).	Regressions, e.g. loss of sphincter control Repression Projection Displacement Aggression Identification Denial and withdrawal Protest behaviour More subtle and passive (refuses to eat, etc.)

Table 3.2 *cont.*

DEVELOPMENTAL STAGE	ANXIETIES	POSSIBLE REACTIONS
	(v) Immobility.	
	(vi) Loss of control (of previously mastered skills).	
	(vii) Body injury and pain.	
Fantasy plays an important part in the preschooler's life and this may give rise to other anxieties.		
4 School children: industry *v.* inferiority	(i) Separation; better understood because of school; but becomes anxious when school friends and family not there.	Protest behaviour less common Boredom Loneliness Frustration Withdrawal Regression
	(ii) Loss of control of previously mastered skills.	Stoicism (may have phobias) Seeks information
	(iii) Body injury and pain. Fears illness, disability, intrusion and death.	Clenches teeth, whines groans Acts bravely Exaggerates
5 Adolescents: identity *v.* role confusion	(i) Loss of control, e.g., identity. (ii) Body injury and pain (altered body image and disfigurement). (iii) Separation from peer group. (iv) Afraid of life and death.	Uncooperativeness Withdrawal Self-assertion Aggression Over-confidence Depression Loneliness Boredom

and anxieties arising from this experience. Crow (1979) noted that children hospitalised for more than two weeks were at risk of disruption to language and development of cognitive skills. Rutter (1972) suggested that hospital could disrupt the bonding/attachment process in infants. Hopkins (1983), reporting on the work of Fagin (1966), points out that hospitalised toddlers who had received only daily

Fig. 3.2 Protest behaviour seen in toddlers and preschool children

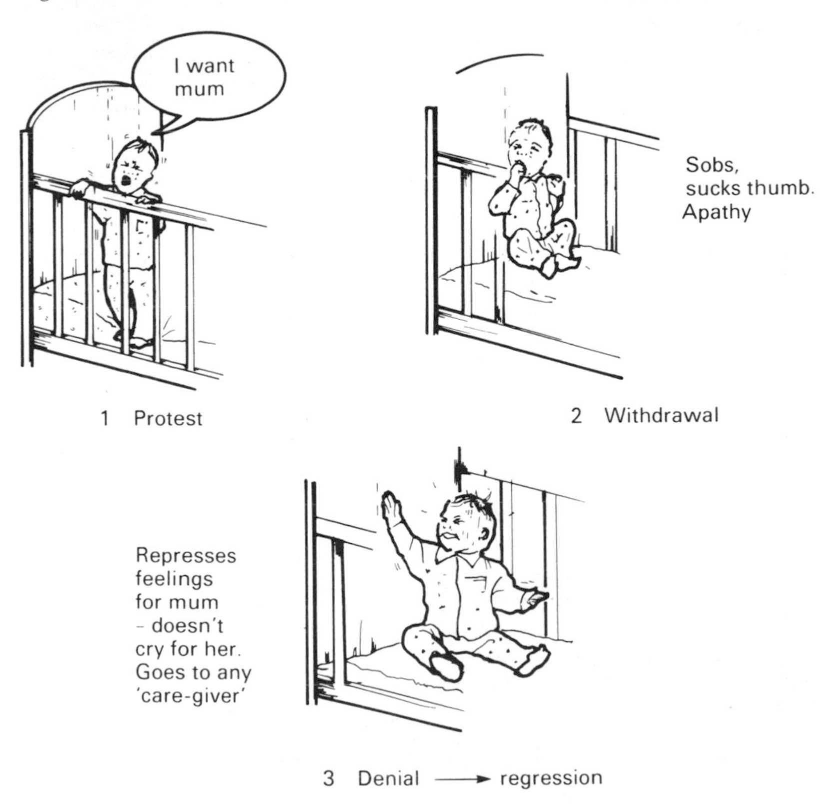

visits from their mothers were seriously behaviourally upset up to one month later, whereas children admitted for minor surgery with their mums showed no significant upset one week after hospital discharge.

Many children take transitional objects (e.g. cuddlies, old pieces of nighties, etc.) to hospital with them. Darbyshire (1985) suggests that work has shown these to be a source of comfort to the child during stress and anxiety.

Finally, in Jolly's (1985) study of children who were asked what it was like to be ill in hospital, those who had never been hospitalised anticipated it to be more stressful than those who had experienced it. Ten-year-old children and those slightly older still experienced stress when separated from their families.

In view of these reports, the need to continue pre-operative preparation for children, consistently to give honest explanations and to welcome and involve parents in the ward, must be high priorities in paediatric care.

PAIN

Recognising pain in children, especially those who are preverbal, is a difficult aspect of paediatric nursing. However, it is important that pain is noted and acted upon quickly to prevent further anxiety and discomfort.

Pain features at different developmental stages

Infants and toddlers (preverbal children)

There is some evidence to suggest that infants feel pain at birth and also that they have different cries for different uncomfortable stimuli. Therefore a cry associated with pain may be different from those associated with hunger or anxiety. When infants respond to a heel prick for collection of blood, it has been noted that they react by withdrawing the foot from the point of stimulus and by spontaneously crying.

For many years, infants have been denied pain relief in the form of analgesia, because it was stated that the nerves had not been completely myelinated and therefore the infant could not feel pain. However, evidence such as reaction to birth and a heel prick dispel such notions.

As infants cannot talk and therefore tell you where it hurts, nurses assume that as they do not complain, they cannot be in pain. The nurse may think that as an infant's pain experience is minimal, he does not feel pain.

Until a child can begin to communicate readily and to localise pain, features other than those given verbally must be sought. This applies also to those in early toddlerhood whose vocabulary is limited.

McGuire and Dizard (1982) suggest the following features could be sought when assessing a child under two for pain: increased irritability; loss of appetite; loss of interest in play. Other features include: a tense body posture; an inability to be comforted; flexing of extremities; head-rolling; lethargy; crying.

Physiological changes are less accurate indicators in the young child, where body processes are developing. Also acute and chronic pain may affect vital signs in different ways.

Preschool, school children and adolescents (verbal children)

It becomes somewhat easier to assess pain in children who can talk. However I am sure we have all met the child who has a 'headache' in his elbow! At least the child knows he has a pain, even if the location terminology is immature.

Despite verbal communication in pain, studies have demonstrated that nurses in paediatric areas are reluctant to give prescribed analgesia, especially if it is ordered 'as necessary'. Nor are children given analgesia as frequently as adults in hospital, and doses can be too small to be effective. McGuire and Dizard (1982) in their research in the USA found that 13:25 children having surgery were not given pain relief throughout the whole of the hospital stay, due to a belief that the young child could tolerate pain. This was based on the study of a group of 5–18 year-olds, results also showing that the younger the child the *lower* the pain tolerance. Nurses and medical staff tended to feel that children 'bounced back', because of their natural resilience.

Williams (1987), in describing the progressive care in the Department of Paediatrics at Nottingham, noted that previous studies (Mather & Mackie 1983) found that children denied pain if an intramuscular injection was the prescribed route of analgesia.

Beales (1982) suggests that children are praised for bravery, but get a negative response when they cry because of pain. If a child yells and screams, he may be labelled a 'softy' or a complainer.

By the preschool and school years, the child attaches pain to a previous or a particular experience, and also knows that external damage to the body is associated with pain. Beales (1982) noted that the worse the injury looks, the more discomfort for the child. How a child reacts to pain may be affected by the explanation and communication he is given. For instance an inflamed knee could mean that the knee was going to catch fire!

There are specific characteristics, however, which the verbal child can show when in pain. McGuire and Dizard (1982) suggest the following features:

— Between the ages of 2 and 7 (Piaget's pre-operational stage (Piaget & Inhelder 1969)) pain illness may be thought of as punishment for being 'bad'.
— Although children can verbalise pain, there may be no connection between pain and medication. Pontious (1982) notes that oral medicine which goes to the stomach is not perceived as taking away a headache!
— The child can use special pain words

(Jerrett & Evans 1986) and can point to pain, i.e. 'where it hurts'.

- He can draw pain on a human body picture.
- He may become restless or change his activity to cope with pain, or may lose his appetite.
- A child may whine or cling to his caregiver or lie quietly on his bed.
- He may wait till parents arrive to express pain.
- Psychosomatic 'fake' pain may appear.
- Vital signs may alter, e.g. in acute pain, pallor, increased pulse and respirations, vomiting, pupil dilatation etc.
- Adolescents may fear becoming addicted to pain medication.

Pain assessment tools

Williams (1987) describes a variety of tools which can be used to assist with assessing a child's pain.

1 The child can point to a colour which denotes pain on a colour scale, e.g. black or red.
2 A linear scale (Fig. 3.3) can also be used (a pain ruler or thermometer). Children must be able to understand the linear scale and be able to understand and verbalise pain.
3 A human body outline for the child to shade the painful area. This may be useful when a child cannot describe pain.

Other assessment tools are:

1 A linear scale with matching words. Adolescents can describe pain and therefore match words, e.g. *severe* or *excruciating* with *the worst pain ever experienced.*
2 Children can point to a series of faces

Fig. 3.3 A linear pain scale

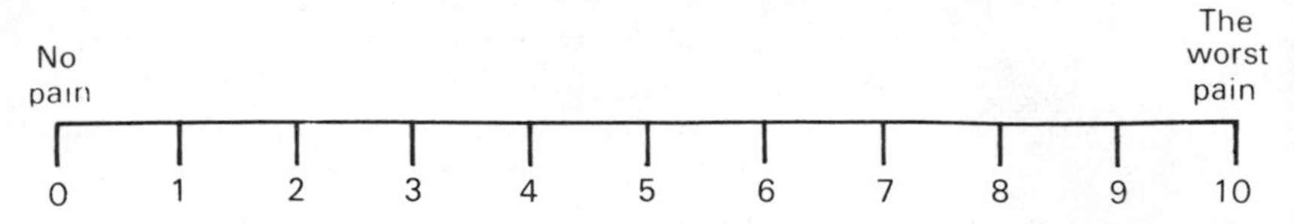

through a range from sad or unhappy to smiling (Fig. 3.4).

3 A pain 'speedometer' may be used, which is similar to a ruler, but uses a clock face or speedometer diagram. The child can show or verbalise the hands either whizzing round the clock or ticking along slowly.
4 Children can act out pain on dolls or toys (see Chapter 9, Expressing sexuality). They can also dress up and act out roles associated with painful episodes, the latter being possible before the event.

Fig. 3.4 Facial expression scale to assess pain. Any variation of faces and words can be used depending on the child's understanding

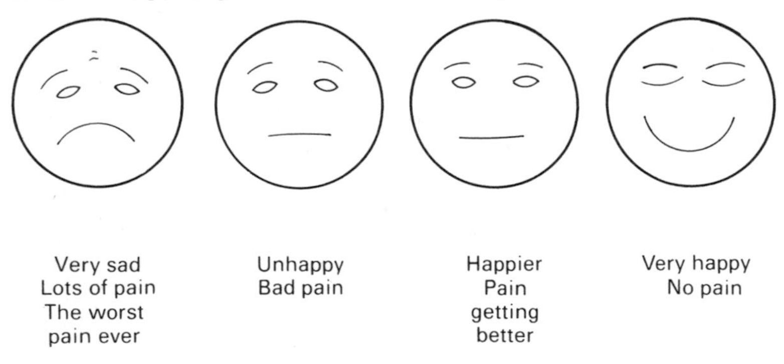

Very sad
Lots of pain
The worst
pain ever

Unhappy
Bad pain

Happier
Pain
getting
better

Very happy
No pain

EXERCISE

With supervision, you could attempt to assess a child's pain using one of the tools described. Alternatively your unit may have its own pain assessment methods.

Jerrett and Evans (1986) used a descriptive study to classify children's pain vocabulary. Some words the children used such as 'weird' and 'sausage' were unclassifiable. Conclusions drawn from this study suggest that children use subjective words such as 'buzzing', or 'like headache', to describe pain, as was to be expected. However they also use affective words, e.g. 'scared' and evaluative words, e.g. 'bad', 'different', 'funny'.

Valley (1984), in a scholarship study, educated staff to use a linear pain assessment scale on children in selected ITU, Burns and Accident & Emergency Departments. Assessments on a 1 to 5 scale ranged from 'sedated, asleep' (1) to 'distressed, causing attention to vital signs' (5). An interim conclusion drawn from the work was that the presence of parents makes a difference to the child's pain. Analgesia prior to procedures and the use of play also contributed to pain relief.

Managing the child's pain: **some practical suggestions**

1 Analgesia must be given regularly as prescribed and constantly assessed for effect. Intramuscular injections should be avoided. Williams (1987) describes the use of local anaesthetic creams before, e.g. venepuncture. Dolls have the cream put on too. The study found the use of Entonox for anaesthesia useful for children over 4 years of age (younger children are not capable of self-administration). Intravenous continuous analgesia infusions can be used (not for neonates). Epidural and subcutaneous infusions are the choice of route of administration in some units.
2 There should be a 'pain-free' area on every

paediatric ward, e.g. the play area. No nursing or medical procedures should be carried out in this area (Williams 1987).

3 Parents should be well informed and listened to about their child's pain. Children should have honest explanations.
4 Play should be used to explain pain both pre- and post the event. Bravery certificates should be given to every child, no matter how they react!
5 Comforting skills should be used as an adjunct to analgesia and not in place of it.

In conclusion, a study by Bradshaw and Zeanah (1986) should be seriously considered when dealing with pain in children. A group of paediatric nurses were asked what criteria they used to identify pain in children. The sample group ranged from those with little experience to those with more than 10 years experience. Following content analysis using the categories shown in Table 3.3 it was noted

Table 3.3 Pain identification used by paediatric nurses (Bradshaw & Zeanah 1986)

CATEGORY CLASSIFICATION	PHYSICAL AND PSYCHOSOCIAL INDICATORS OF PAIN IN CHILDREN
Oral expression	Cries, groaning
Verbal communication	Hurts, wants pain relief
Facial expression	Wrinkled forehead, grimace
Body language	Posturing, holds body, tense
Affect	Withdrawal, depression, anxiety, irritability
Physiological changes	Vital signs, colour, nausea, vomiting
Nurses' judgement	Consideration of time and type of procedure, knowledge of child, time of last medication, stage of illness
Parents' assessment	Asks for relief of child's pain
Relief action	Rocking, comforting

that the more experienced nurses used body language and oral expression mainly to assess pain, followed by the child's affect and physiological changes and parental assessment.

The knowledge of the child and his previous experiences were not assessed. No distinction was made between acute and chronic pain indicators.

REFERENCES

BEALES, J. G. 1982. Suffer the little children. *Nursing Mirror,* **155**(11), 58–59.

BRADSHAW, C. & ZEANAH, P. D. 1986. Paediatric nurses' assessment of pain in children. *Journal of Paediatric Nursing,* (5), 314–22.

CROW, R. 1979. Sensory Deprivation in Children. *Nursing Times,* **75**(6), 229–233.

DARBYSHIRE, P. 1985. Happiness is an old blanket. *Nursing Times,* **81**(10), 40–41.

DARBYSHIRE, P. 1985. Life without Teddy. *Nursing Times,* **81**(11), 44–46.

DAVIE, R., BUTLER, N. & GOLDSTEIN, H. 1972. *From Birth to Seven.* The second report of the National Development Study. Longman, London.

FAGIN, C. 1966. *The effects of maternal attendance during hospitalisation on the post hospital behaviour of young children.* F. A. Davis, Philadelphia.

FOULGER, K. 1985. *Wiggly's Story.* Bristol Royal Hospital for Sick Children.

FRADD, E. 1987. A Special Case. ABPN Spotlight on Children. *Nursing Times,* **83**(51), 55.

HAWTHORN, P. 1974. *Nurse, I want my Mummy.* RCN Research Series, London.

HOPKINS, J. 1983. Hospitalisation: 1. The Psychotherapist's View. ABPN Spotlight on Children. *Nursing Times,* **79**(42), 42–45.

JERRETT, M. & EVANS, K. 1986. Children's pain vocabulary. *Journal of Advanced Nursing,* **11**, 403–408.

JOLLY, J. 1985. Child Health: Timmy goes to hospital. *Nursing Times,* **81**(13), 27–30.

LEWER, H. & ROBERTSON, L. 1987. *Care of the Child,* 2nd Edn. Essentials of Nursing Series. Macmillan, London.

McGUIRE, L. & DIZARD, S. 1982. Managing Pain in the Young Patient. *Nursing*, **82** (August), 52–55.
MATHER, L. & MACKIE, J. 1983. The Incidence of Post Operative Pain in Children. *Pain*, **15**, 271–282.
MINISTRY OF HEALTH. 1959. *The Welfare of Children in Hospital*. Report of the Platt Committee. HMSO, London.
PIAGET, J. & INHELDER, B. 1969. *The Psychology of the Child*. Routledge & Kegan Paul, London.
PONTIOUS, S. 1982. Practical Piaget, helping children understand. *American Journal of Nursing*, (January), 114–117.
ROBERTSON, J. 1953. Some Responses of Young Children to Loss of Maternal Care. *Nursing Times*, **49**, 382–386.
RODIN, J. 1983. Will this hurt? *Preparing children for hospital and medical procedures*. RCN Research Series, London.
ROPER, N., LOGAN, W. & TIERNEY, A. J. 1985. *The Elements of Nursing*, 2nd Edn. Churchill Livingstone, Edinburgh.
RUTTER, M. 1972. *Maternal Deprivation Reassessed*. Penguin Educational, London.
VALLEY, L. 1984. *Interim report on Pain in Children*. (Unpublished) ABPN/Portex Scholarship Study.
WILLIAMS, J. (1987). Managing Paediatric Pain. *Nursing Times*, **83**(36), 36–39.

FURTHER READING

ALTHAEA BOOKS FOR CHILDREN. 1973–1974. *Going to the Doctor. Visiting the Dentist. Going into Hospital. Dinosaur Publications.*
BONNER, M. 1986. Can my friend go with me? *Nursing Times*, **82**(40), 75–76.
BOWLBY, J. 1965. *Child care and the growth of love*. Penguin, Harmondsworth.
DAY, A. 1987. Can mummy come too? ABPN Spotlight on Children. *Nursing Times*, **83**(51), 51–52.
GLASPER, A. & DEWAR, A. 1987. Help or Hazard? ABPN Spotlight on Children. *Nursing Times*, **83**(51), 53–54.
JEPSON, M. E. 1983. *Community Child Health*. Hodder & Stoughton, London.
MELZACK, R & WALL, P. 1982. *The challenge of pain*. Penguin, Harmondsworth.

MITCHELL, R. G. (Ed.). 1980. *Child health in the community*, 2nd Ed. Churchill Livingstone, Edinburgh.

4 Breathing

The importance of being able to breathe properly, and take in oxygen to perfuse the tissues and the ability of the heart to circulate blood to vital organs, are of priority in nursing both children and adults.

This chapter considers how healthy breathing can be promoted throughout childhood and how to assess the child who is admitted to hospital with breathing difficulties. Nursing care plans are used to illustrate illnesses which bring children to hospital, namely a toddler with croup and an adolescent in sickle cell crisis.

Health promotion and education

Infants and toddlers

Maintenance of the airway especially in infancy should consider the following factors:

— Infants do not coordinate mouth breathing if their nose becomes blocked. A gag reflex is present from birth, however the infant can still obstruct by being unable to nose breathe. Ensure the nose is cleaned frequently, especially before and after feeds, with cotton wool (ensure wisps of wool are not inhaled).

— Infants should not have a pillow until after the first year and then this is dependent on their development. Catnets should be used on prams when outside.

— After feeding, ensure 'wind' is brought up

and that there is no milk in the mouth. Lie the infant propped on his side; the use of the prone position for infants is inadvisable, as they are unable to lift their heads from the mattress and may bury their noses.

- Seek advice if the infant acquires a cold. The Health Clinic, health visitor or general practitioner may be involved.
- Ensure that the immunisation programme is commenced when advised, to protect against childhood infectious diseases. Infants' immunity to any diseases is minimal until the immune system develops fully and they come into contact with foreign organisms. A poor heat-regulating mechanism can contribute to a predisposition to acquiring infectious illness.
- Toddlers, although more able to maintain their airway both physiologically and immunologically, are at risk of ingestion and inhalation. A toddler can inhale a peanut or poke small objects in his nose and mouth, so vigilance must be maintained.

Preschool and school children and adolescents

- Continuation of the immunisation programme both preschool and in adolescence may protect the child from debilitating infectious illness (see p. 18). Tuberculosis may be prevented or detected with the screening programme during adolescence. Rubella vaccine for adolescent girls is given to prevent harmful effects on the foetus should a subsequent pregnancy occur.
- Glue-sniffing and smoking may be started during school days, either through peer pressure or following the role model of

parents, especially where smoking is concerned. The school health service should provide health education on such topics (Hanson 1987).

Developmental aspects

The respiratory organs

The lungs and air passages are proportionally smaller in diameter and shorter in length than the adult's. The nose is short and squat, with a depressed bridge. The posterior choanae are small and can become easily occluded. The overall distance from the nasopharynx to the lungs is short.

The infant can sneeze, cough, gag and swallow, however an excessive amount of milk or fluids will cause a problem which cannot be dealt with by these reflexes. Premature infants are born without surfactant, which lines the alveoli and encourages expansion of the air-sacs after birth. These infants are at risk of Respiratory Distress Syndrome (RDS).

The cardiovascular organs

The heart size of the young child is proportionally larger and occupies more space in the pleural cavity. The apex of the heart is located at the level of the 3rd and 4th intercostal spaces, lateral to the midclavicular line.

The blood vessels, whose diameter is regulated by the autonomic nervous system, do not respond as in the adult, because of immaturity of the nervous system. The circulating blood volume in the newborn infant is 270 millilitres. The distribution of fluid in the cells and tissues differs from that in the older child (see p. 107)

CHECK LIST

Assessment of the child's breathing and blood circulation

In an emergency maintain airway and seek nursing and medical assistance, after checking breathing and pulse.

Cardiopulmonary resuscitation

1 *Ventilation of the airway: infants*
Clear mouth and nose of mucus or vomit with finger or suction. Extend neck with hand or a rolled towel or nappy under the infant's shoulders.
Take a breath and tightly seal your mouth over the infant's mouth and nose.
Blow a small amount of air gently into the airway.
Always remove your mouth from the infant's in between ventilations.

2 *Ventilation of the airway: older children*
As for infants, except that the nose should be pinched and ventilation takes place through the mouth only. A larger quantity of air is necessary; expansion of the chest will indicate effective volume.

3 *External cardiac massage*
Ensure the child is on a firm support for effective cardiac massage.

For infants, two fingers on the chest wall or both thumbs placed on top of each other with the hands wrapped around the chest will provide sufficient compression. The heel of one hand may be used for the young child, whilst in older children both hands are used.

Non-emergency assessment

1 Ask parents the history of the child's breathing difficulties and note the observations the parents have made on their child.
2 Look at the whole picture; is the child restless, lethargic, crying, in pain or dehydrated?

Table 4.1 External cardiac massage for children (Weller 1986)

CHILD SIZE	MASSAGE RATE	RATIO OF COMPRESSIONS TO VENTILATIONS
Small infant	100–120/min	3:1
Larger infant	80–100/min	3:1
Small child	80–100/min	4–5:1
Larger child	60–80/min	5:1

3 What is the child's colour? Infants often turn grey when ill, rather than the bluish colour associated with cyanosis in older children and adults.
4 Is breathing noisy, e.g. mucusy, or with stridor due to spasm or oedema?
5 Is breathing laboured, irregular (infants often pause at intervals between breathing and asthmatic children have difficulty expiring)? Does the chest move equally?
6 Is breathing regular, of sufficient depth, using accessory muscles?
7 Is the pulse of a good rhythm and volume and is it regular?
8 Is the blood pressure recordable?

CARE PLAN

A toddler with croup

Freddie Thompson was a normally lively two-year-old, who lived with his mother and father in a small terraced house on the outskirts of a town. Freddie had no brothers or sisters and had started to attend a toddler club with his mother, to get used to meeting and playing with other children. When he developed a

Table 4.2 Developmental changes in observations of respirations, pulse and blood pressure

DEVELOPMENTAL STAGE	RESPIRATIONS PER MINUTE RANGE	AVERAGE	PULSE PER MINUTE RANGE	AVERAGE	BLOOD PRESSURE mmHg
Newborn	30–50	35	70–170 (apex)	120	80/50
Infant 1 year	26–40	30	80–160 (apex)	120	90/61
Toddler 2 years	20–30	25	80–130 (radial)	110	95/61
Preschool child 4 years	20–30	23	80–120 (radial)	100	99/65
School child 8 years	18–24	20	70–110 (radial)	90	105/57
Adolescent 15 years	12–20	17	60–110 (radial)	80 girls; 75 boys	121/61

cold, his mother thought he had acquired it from the toddlers at the club. However, by the next day Freddie had noisy crowing breathing and was very lethargic. His parents rang the GP who advised that he be admitted to hospital immediately (see Chapter 3).

Definition of croup Croup is a congestion and swelling of the vocal cords together with spasm of the larynx and laryngeal muscles. The cause is usually viral, such as the respiratory syncytial virus and the onset may be either gradual or acute. In the early stages it is difficult to diagnose whether the 'croupy breathing', is due to a simple laryngitis, laryngo–tracheo–bronchitis, or to a foreign body or acute epiglottitis. The latter is a paediatric emergency.

Predisposition to croup Children between the ages of 6 months and 2 years are most at risk and in the winter months particularly.

Clinical features of croup Clinical features may either appear acutely or with the gradual onset of a cold, low grade pyrexia, hoarseness and crowing inspiratory stridor.

ADMISSION TO HOSPITAL

On admission to the ward, Freddie was distressed as he could not breathe easily, or speak or eat without becoming extremely breathless. He and his mum were shown to a cot and Freddie was content to sit in it, as long as his mother cuddled him. The nurse was quick to take details about Freddie and commence his prescribed treatment.

Care plan for Freddie during the acute phase

PROBLEM 1

Problem	*Aims of nursing care*
Hoarse, 'crowing' and difficult inspiratory breathing due to laryngeal spasm and oedema. Inability to speak properly.	Maintain Freddie's airway and promote oxygenation of the tissues. Encourage Freddie's parents to communicate with staff about Freddie.

NURSING CARE

Ensure emergency equipment is available (suction and oxygen). Place Freddie in a humidity tent and administer humidified air or oxygen, as prescribed by the doctor. Humidification decreases the swelling around the larynx, thereby relieving noisy and difficult inspiratory breathing.

Ensure Freddie is not separated from his parents and let him adopt a position of comfort in the cot, preferably upright.

Monitor and record pulse and respiratory rates half-hourly and note his colour.

Administer prescribed medications to promote rest and prevent bacterial infection.

Involve the physiotherapist if secretions are obstructing the airway.

EVALUATION

Respiratory rate, effort and Freddie's colour will indicate effectiveness of care and treatment. Cessation of stridor will occur when laryngeal swelling has decreased and Freddie can be taken out of his tent.

PROBLEM 2

Problem
Frightened child due to emergency admission, difficulty with breathing and being nursed in a humidity tent. Also frightened due to limited mobility.

Aim of nursing care
Prevent anxiety and later post-hospital behaviour.

NURSING CARE

Ensure parents are welcomed and informed about their child's admission. Offer a place for them to stay and inform them about hospital routine and environment. By keeping the child and his parents together, the sense of trust and security should be maintained. This is especially essential during the toddler years when a child can see a parent is not by their bedside, but cannot understand where the parent has gone.

Give Freddie comforting toys, especially any favourites from home. Cuddly blankets and 'special' items are invaluable when the child is sick to provide continuity from home. Toddlers interpret limits to mobilising as punishment, so it is vital both that Freddie is safe in his tent, and that he can be picked up and cuddled by his parents.

EVALUATION

Freddie's general attitude to parents and staff will indicate whether he is less frightened. The long-term effects of hospitalisation will not be noted until Freddie returns home. (Hopkins 1983; Muller *et al.* 1986).

PROBLEM 3

Problem	*Aim of nursing care*
Low grade pyrexia: 37.5°C	Reduce temperature gradually to within normal range of 35.9°C–36.7°C (axilla).

NURSING CARE

Record Freddie's temperature hourly and report if it increases above 37.5°C. Freddie is at risk of febrile convulsions, therefore he may be prescribed an anti-pyretic medicine to reduce his temperature.

Being nursed in a humidity tent can cause Freddie to become agitated and restless, making him hot and sweaty; the temperature within the tent can become very warm. Dress Freddie in minimal cotton clothing and a nappy, and keep him clean, dry and cool; he may need a gentle wash to make him comfortable.

EVALUATION

Freddie's temperature remained at 37.5°C for 4 hours and then reduced to 36.9°C by the evening.

PROBLEM 4

Problem
Dry, furred mouth and dry skin, decreased urine output, general lethargy; due to increased respirations, lack of fluid intake and pyrexia.

Aim of nursing care
Maintain state of hydration; ensure Freddie does not become dehydrated.

NURSING CARE

Give parents fluids to offer Freddie and ensure these are taken half-hourly. Record all fluid intake and urine output on a fluid balance chart.

Observe Freddie's skin turgor, especially the soft tissues around the eyes.

EVALUATION

Initially Freddie did not want to drink, however his state of hydration was good and did not necessitate commencing an intravenous infusion. As his breathing rate slowed to within the normal range he drank from a teacher beaker.

PARENTAL EDUCATION

Admission to hospital for croup is usually short, sometimes lasting only 24 hours. Children are unlikely to need a further admission for this illness.

Freddie's parents need to be reassured that complications are unlikely and warned to expect a few changes in his behaviour following hospitalisation.

Some children with croup can be treated at home by sitting with them in a steamy room, often the bathroom, until the stridor subsides (longer than 10 minutes and the GP should be notified).

Freddie's antibiotics should be continued and he should not return to the toddler club until these are completed and his mother feels he has recovered.

CARE PLAN

An adolescent in sickle cell crisis

Florence Mercury, aged fifteen had been diagnosed as having sickle cell anaemia at the age of two. As Florence was of West Indian origin, her parents, although upset, were not entirely shocked, knowing that sickle cell anaemia is relatively common amongst the West Indian population. As many years had elapsed since her first diagnosis and Florence had suffered numerous sickle cell crises, she knew what to expect each time a crisis occurred. This made her somewhat anxious and insecure, especially as schooling was regularly interrupted because of frequent periods in hospital. Florence had two sisters, Martha and Jo, and one brother, Bradley. When Florence was first diagnosed as having sickle cell anaemia the whole family were also tested. Martha and Jo were found to have sickle cell trait (i.e. they were carriers but not affected with the disease).

Fig. 4.1 Inheritance of sickle cell in Florence's family. (You may need to check your knowledge of genetic inheritance in your anatomy and physiology textbook)

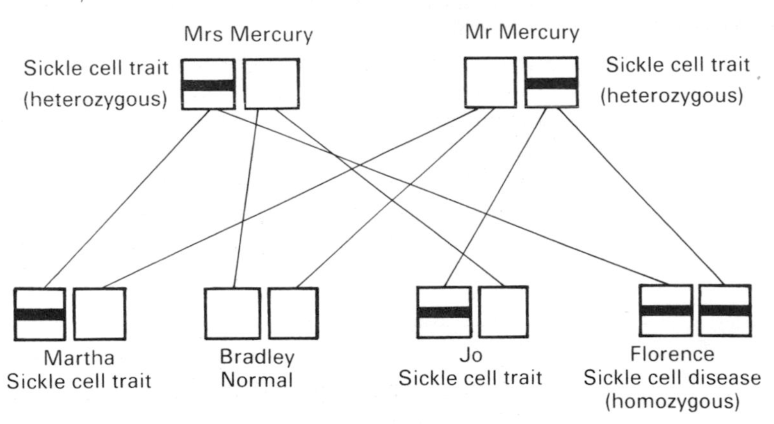

Definition of sickle cell anaemia and crisis Sickle cell anaemia is an inherited disease, where the red blood cells contain Haemoglobin S (HbS) and there is a reduced O_2 uptake. Some HbS may persist in early infancy; however infants normally revert to adult haemoglobin (HbA) after the first few months of life. Sickle cell anaemia may be detected by blood electrophoresis after three months of age. The genetic deformity causes the red blood cells to adopt a sickle shape at times of low oxygen tension and when the pH of the body is low.

The sickle cells agglutinate in small blood vessels such as the kidneys, joints and spleen and this causes extreme pain and decreased tissue oxygenation. During a 'sickling' episode, the child is said to be in crisis.

Predisposition to sickle cell crisis Factors which predispose the child to a crisis are: hypoxia (e.g. caused by air travel or during an operation); infection; dehydration; physical exercise; trauma.

ADMISSION TO HOSPITAL

Florence arrived on the children's ward, where she was well known, with severe pain in her knee, breathless and very anxious. Observations of pulse recorded a rate of 120 beats per minute, her respirations were 28 per minute and there were indications of cyanosis (lips and nail beds).

An attempt was made to measure Florence's pain with a pain ruler (see p. 67). However, she was too distraught for this to be effective and in medical opinion, needed a strong analgesic on admission, to relieve pain, as well as being placed on bed rest. Mrs Mercury accompanied Florence into the ward, the other children being at school. The details of the onset of the crisis were taken by the doctor from Mrs Mercury, who then needed to sit quietly by Florence's bedside with a cup of tea.

Care plan for Florence during the acute period of sickle cell crisis

PROBLEM 1

Problem
Breathlessness and poor colour due to lowered oxygen uptake by sickle cells and subsequent acidosis (see Problem 4).

Aims of nursing care
Relieve breathlessness and reduce respirations to within normal limits (12–20/min).

NURSING CARE

Place Florence in a quiet bay in the ward, on bed rest in a position of comfort. Administer oxygen via a face mask as prescribed by the doctor.

Explain all that you do to Florence and her mother, as relief of anxiety may help lower respirations.

Assist the doctor in commencing an infusion (if not already done in the Accident & Emergency Department). Grouping and cross-matching of Florence's blood will have been done on previous admissions, and as soon as possible a blood transfusion will be commenced.

Observe Florence half-hourly for pulse rate, respiratory rate and colour and hourly temperature. Ensure the transfusion runs to time and that the cannula site is not leaking or inflamed. Check that Florence does not become more breathless or have loin or back pain, a pyrexia or rash. These clinical features may be a reaction to the transfusion and prompt reporting and action must be taken.

The prescription of oxygen and blood transfusion will provide the body with correctly formed red blood cells, which will be able to take up oxygen more readily and therefore reduce breathlessness and improve colour.

EVALUATION

A reduction in Florence's respiratory rate, colour and pulse rate will indicate the problems are reducing. The Hb level will only be returned to the normal 6–7G/100 ml seen in many children with sickle cell anaemia.

PROBLEM 2

Problem
Severe pain and swelling in left knee and probable pain in abdomen – due to agglutination of sickle cells in fine blood capillaries.

Aim of nursing care
Relieve and control pain within a few hours of admission.

NURSING CARE

Administer intramuscular (IM) strong analgesia (the doctor may give intravenous (IV) analgesia) and observe for effects and side effects. A pain ruler can be used after the initial dose of analgesia has had effect (see p. 67).

Let Florence position herself comfortably in bed; her leg may need supporting on a firm pillow. Talk and comfort Florence, use gentle touch and encourage Mrs Mercury to be involved. Control of pain will lessen anxiety and breathlessness and prevent complications such as stiffness of the knee joint, when Florence starts to weight bear.

EVALUATION

Check when Florence's pain subsides following analgesia and note this down. Ensure that pain relief will be given before pain recurs. Note how Florence is lying in bed and any other clues which may show she has pain.

PROBLEM 3

Problem
Anxiety due to emergency admission, pain, breathlessness and missing school.

Aim of nursing care
Relieve anxiety by careful explanation and maintain contact with family, friends and school.

NURSING CARE

Florence is 15 years old and has had sickle cell crisis before, she knows what treatment and care to expect and this can heighten her anxiety. Explanation of all procedures is vital and Florence needs time to talk about her worries, which may include a fear of dying. Family should have free access for visiting and Florence's friends should be kept in contact with her. The school can be phoned up and if the hospital admission is likely to be extended, then a school teacher may visit Florence in the paediatric ward. (This will be a subsequent priority.)

EVALUATION

Florence will appear more relaxed and able to communicate with nursing staff. Vital signs may also reflect a lessening of anxiety.

PROBLEM 4

Problem	*Aim of nursing care*
(p) Nausea; (p) vomiting; dry skin; dry mouth. Decreased urine output including bilirubinuria due to decreased fluid volume, acidosis and agglutination/ haemolysis.	Prevent Florence becoming dehydrated by preventing nausea and vomiting.

NURSING CARE

Florence has an intravenous cannula *in situ* initially for the blood transfusion. Intravenous fluids will be given following the transfusion to prevent further acidosis and dehydration. If Florence is nauseous an intramuscular (IM) anti-emetic may be prescribed and administered. She will need two-hourly mouth care and ice to suck. A vomit bowel and tissues should be on her locker. Once nausea and vomiting subside, hourly clear fluids should be offered and as Florence improves, a light and attractive diet given.

Careful observation of Florence's skin state, oral cavity and urine output should be made and recorded. An intake and output chart should be maintained.

Urine should be tested for blood, urobilinogen and bilirubin. Once the agglutinated sickle cells begin to haemolyse, the breakdown products, i.e. bilirubin, may be excreted in the urine and haematuria may also occur. All urine results should be recorded.

EVALUATION

Maintenance of a fluid balance chart will indicate if Florence is in fluid balance. Observation of skin and oral cavity as well as urine output will indicate her state of hydration. Alterations in urinary constituents may indicate the stage of the crisis.

PROBLEM 5

Problem	*Aim of nursing care*
(p) Raised temperature, due to alteration in fluid and electrolyte balance. Primarily due to infection which may have caused the sickle cell crisis.	Reduce temperature to within normal range, 35.9°C–36.7°C (axilla)

NURSING CARE

Florence will need an hourly temperature recording, taken per axilla as she is breathless. A pyrexia must be reported and an antipyretic may be prescribed and administered. Encouraging fluids may also assist with temperature reduction. Swabs may be taken from the nose and throat and any other specimens which the doctor may order, to assist with the diagnosis of the predisposing factors. Antibiotics may be prescribed.

If Florence does become pyrexial, she should have minimum clothing on and over her body and a fan by the beside, to cool the air around her. Tepid sponging should be done only if ordered by a senior member of the nursing staff or by the doctor. The procedure must be done with caution, ensuring the temperature does not fall more than 1°C in one minute, as a sudden fall in temperature may cause shock.

Infection is one of the predisposing factors of sickle cell crisis.

EVALUATION

Monitoring of temperature will indicate Florence's response to treatment.

SUBSEQUENT CARE

Once Florence is not breathless, cyanosed or in severe pain she will be able to mobilise. The administration of blood and oxygen are measures usually taken during the acute period. An intravenous infusion may be continued until Florence is well hydrated and blood electrolytes are satisfactory. Pain relief will be adjusted according to the degree of pain and the effect of the medications. An oral analgesic may be necessary for several days. If antibiotics are commenced, the course must be completed.

Florence will go home when pain has subsided, blood electrolytes and urinary results are within normal limits and when she does not have a pyrexia.

PATIENT EDUCATION

It is important that Florence leads as near normal a life as possible. The life span of children with sickle cell anaemia is shortened and the effects of repeated crises can lead to joint and limb deformities. Frequent transfusions of blood can lead to heart failure and haemosiderosis (laying down of iron in the tissues). More recently, concern has been heightened about receiving blood products because of human immunodeficiency viruses (HIV) transmitted in blood products. All donor blood is now routinely screened for HIV.

Florence should return to school as soon as she is able and with the help of the school medical team, the school teacher, the district nurse and, of course, her family she should be helped to maintain her health. This includes no severe sudden exercise, avoiding infection, having regular dental checkups and generally caring for her skin properly. Air travel should not be attempted until medical advice has been sought.

Florence will need to have someone with whom she can discuss her worries, her future and the progress of her disease. The Sickle Cell Association is a support group for parents and children who have the disease.

REFERENCES

HANSON, L. 1987. No Longer the Nit Lady. *Nursing Times*, **83**(22), 30–32.

HOPKINS, J. 1983. Hospitalisation. 1. The psychotherapist's view. ABPN Spotlight on Children. *Nursing Times* **79**(42), 42–45.

MULLER, D. J., HARRIS, P. J. & WATTLEY, L. 1986. *Nursing Children: Psychology, Research and Practice*. Lippincott Nursing Series. Harper & Row, London.

WELLER, B. F. 1986. *The Lippincott Manual of Paediatric Nursing*. Lippincott Nursing Series. Harper & Row, London.

WHALEY, L. F. & WONG, D. L. 1983. *Nursing Care of Infants and Sick Children*, 2nd Edn. Mosby, St Louis.

5 Maintaining body temperature

Febrile convulsion is a seizure associated with a raised temperature, usually above 38.5°C. There is a familial predisposition to febrile convulsions.

This chapter considers how maintenance of body temperature may be achieved during early childhood and how to assess a child admitted to hospital with a pyrexia. Febrile convulsion is discussed. A brief care plan is included, to illustrate the principles of caring for children admitted with a pyrexia.

Health promotion and education

Infants, toddlers and school children

Maintenance of a constant body temperature should consider the following factors:

— Infants have a large surface area to body weight ratio, so heat loss can be greater. Fingers and toes, as well as the head which is large in comparison to the body, can become cold easily. Bonnets, mittens and bootees are essential for young infants. Layers of cotton clothing should be worn and the infant covered with a sheet and blanket or a light quilt. Wrapping the infant up firmly not only keeps him warm, but gives a feeling of security.

— Infants are unable to regulate their body temperature as adults can, due to immaturity of the heat regulating mechanism, as well as developmental immaturity. Therefore keep the environmental temperature warm; but do not put an infant in front of the fire, wrapped up in blankets as he will overheat and this may cause a febrile convulsion and/or dehydration.

— Do put infants outside in the garden, unless the outside temperature is extremely hot or cold; protection from strong sun or wind should be provided.
— Toddlers, although more able to maintain body temperature due to physical development, are still at risk of febrile convulsions. They also become involved playing and forget they are cold. This often happens to school children who rush to play outside, forgetting the need to dress in relation to environmental temperature.
— School teachers should ensure children are warmly dressed before going out to play during breaks between lessons.

Developmental aspects

Infants have a high metabolic rate and therefore their temperature may be higher than the normal stated in Table 5.1. There is a developmental inability to regulate body temperature in young infants, because of immaturity of the hypothalamus and autonomic nervous system. Infants neither sweat nor shiver, both of which are means of losing or conserving heat. Neither do they alter their peripheral blood vessels to vasodilate (lose heat) or constrict (conserve heat).

It is also possible that the normal circadian rhythm is not established and fluctuations in temperature in keeping with this 24-hour cycle may not be seen.

The surface area of the infant available for heat loss is great in comparison with body weight, which is small. The head represents one third to a quarter of body length and is a source of heat loss.

Inability to regulate the body temperature may persist through the toddler years, up to the age of three. Infants and young children are at risk of febrile convulsions up to this age.

CHECK LIST

Assessment of the child's body temperature

During a febrile convulsion: maintain the child's airway by placing him on his side. Suction may be necessary if saliva occludes the airway. Ensure the child is safe and cannot roll out of bed, or harm part of his body on furniture or equipment. Stay with the child until the convulsion subsides, having gained assistance from a paediatric nurse. Time the length of the convulsion and the nature of it and report to nursing staff. Record the child's temperature and maintain a half-hourly chart. Following the convulsion, the child may be given an antipyretic.

It is important to note that **febrile convulsion** is *not* an **epileptic convulsion** and if parents are present, to ensure they know that the convulsion is related to a high body temperature.

Assessment of a child with a pyrexia

1 Ask parents how long the child has had a pyrexia and any observations they have made. The child may have had a runny nose, a cough, earache or abdominal pain, nausea and vomiting – all features which are important to note in assisting with the diagnosis.

2 Does the child look as if he is in pain, if so where? Is the child crying or restless?

3 Is the child dehydrated? Look at the skin turgor, especially at the groins, limbs and around the eyes. The oral cavity may be dry and the tongue furred.

The anterior fontanelle in infants under 18 months is a useful indication of the state of hydration. If it is depressed it can mean the infant is dehydrated (see p. 111, Chapter 6, Eating and drinking).

4 Are there any discharges from eyes, nose, ears, mouth or from the umbilicus or genito–urinary tract. Urine may smell offensive and look cloudy if an infection is present.

5 Has he been sick? Is the child hot and flushed; if so is the skin dry or moist? Does he look grey and shocked, i.e. peritonitis?

6 Is there any evidence of trauma to the body, such as burns or scalds?

7 Are there any rashes on the body? (Childhood infections or illnesses, such as measles or chicken pox.) If so, how is the rash distributed over the skin?

8 Has the child had any medications or immunisations recently?

Recording body temperature

Table 5.1 Range of body temperature for all age groups

Oral	36.4–37.4°C
Rectal	36.2–37.8°C
Axilla	35.9–36.7°C

Oral and per axilla: For young children under 5 years old, it is safest to record axillary temperature. Mentally handicapped children may always need their temperature taken *per axilla*.

Rectal: This method of temperature measurement is used in critical circumstances and for very small infants. Care must be taken not to damage the rectal mucosa or to cause psychological damage.

Variations between recordings in the different body cavities may be noted in Table 5.1. Evidence suggests (Goodall 1986) that oral recordings should be taken over four minutes and *per axilla* recording for longer to obtain an accurate measurement.

Oral measurements reflect the core body temperature, whereas axillary recordings reflect only the skin surface temperature.

CARE PLAN

A toddler with a pyrexia

Toddlers admitted to hospital with a pyrexia may have acquired this because of any of the following: infection, e.g. meningitis; inflammatory diseases; dehydration, e.g. gastroenteritis or pyloric stenosis; drugs; toxins; tumours.

Pyrexias may be low-grade, i.e. 37.5°C, often associated with appendicitis, or a higher grade pyrexia, often above 38–39°C, associated with meningitis, for example.

Care plan during the acute phase

PROBLEM

Problem
Raised body temperature due to one of the above causes.

Aims of nursing care
Gradually, reduce temperature to within normal limits, 35.9–36.7°C. Prevent a febrile convulsion.

NURSING CARE

Observe toddler carefully for conscious level, behaviour changes and for febrile convulsions. Report any of the above immediately. Record hourly axillary temperatures. Dress the toddler only in a cotton gown and nappy. If hyperpyrexial, he may feel more comfortable without any clothes, except for a light cotton sheet placed over him. A fan, suitably placed away from the cot side, may cool the surrounding air. Cool washes should be used with great caution (see p. 88 Chapter 4, Breathing: An adolescent in sickle cell crisis).

By exposing the toddler's skin to the atmosphere, the principles of convection, radiation and evaporation are utilised, to increase heat loss from the body.

An antipyretic will be prescribed and administered and fluid intake increased. Until recently the medicine of choice was aspirin, however, following recent reports linking aspirin with Reye's Syndrome, this medicine is not recommended for children.

Because the toddler has an increased basal metabolic rate (BMR) his requirements for fluids also increase. If he shows signs of dehydration, an intravenous infusion may be commenced.

At all times, the toddler should be with his family, who will be able to comfort him and encourage fluids, as well as preventing emotional distress which could precipitate a further pyrexia.

EVALUATION

A return to normal temperature, no behaviour changes, febrile convulsions or dehydration are the evaluation factors.

PATIENT EDUCATION

Utilising the information on page 91, teach parents how to maintain a constant body temperature for the young child. It is also useful to ensure they know what action to take should their child have a febrile convulsion in the future.

FURTHER READING

GOODALL, C. 1986. Heat Trials. *Nursing Times*, **82**(8), 46–47.

BOYLAN, A. & BROWN, P. 1985. Temperature: Student Observations. *Nursing Times*, **81**(16), 36–40.

6 Eating and drinking

This chapter considers the changing nutritional requirements of children and the development of the social skills associated with eating and drinking. The distribution of fluid and electrolytes in body compartments differs during early infancy from later childhood and regulation of fluid intake and output is critical for infants. The alimentary tract grows and matures and teeth appear in the first year, so changing the child's nutritional requirements.

To illustrate problems arising from eating and drinking, a care plan for an infant with pyloric stenosis is included. At the other end of the childhood age spectrum is an obese adolescent whose care plan you are encouraged to complete.

Health promotion and education

Infants: breast or bottle feeding

The choice of breast or bottle is entirely individual to each family. Whilst maternal grandmother's influence may play a significant role in the choice, it should be remembered that maternal health and socio-economic status may be strong influences on which method is chosen. The mother should be helped to maintain a good fluid and nutritional status for the infant and for herself.

Breast feeding

As soon as the infant is born, he may be put to the breast to suckle. The suckling reflex is present at birth and the close contact between mother and infant during breast feeding is thought to assist the 'bonding' process.

Breast milk comes into the breast partly by the stimulation of sucking by the infant and partly under the control of hormones, mainly oxytocin and prolactin. Milk is not ejected through the milk ducts until around the third post-natal day. However, colostrum, a protein-rich substance, appears as a thick watery substance and is high in immunoglobin A (IgA), therefore assisting the vulnerable immune status of the infant. Even when breast feeding is not to be continued, suckling in the first few days will give the infant valuable immunological protection through colostrum.

It takes time to establish a breast feeding routine, but this usually revolves around demand feeding. When the infant is awake he is usually hungry and this coincides with a three- to four-hourly pattern. At first, suckling should only be for a few minutes on each breast. Proper fixation on the nipple is essential to ensure the infant takes in milk and not air and also that the mother does not get sore nipples. Taking advantage of the rooting reflex (see p. 136) may help fixation. Over a period of time, the length of breast feeding will increase up to 15 minutes per breast.

The infant is weighed regularly at the Health Clinic or on the health visitor's scales. Approximately 200 gm per week should be gained for the first three months, dropping to 120 gm per week from three to twelve months. This assists the infant to grow along an acceptable growth centile (see p. 134).

Not every mother finds breast feeding comes naturally, and many need privacy and encouragement. Social acceptability about breast feeding varies, with some institutions providing mother and baby rooms and ensuring mothers have time to leave work regularly, whilst others do not encourage breast feeding mothers to return to work.

Because of the physical involvement and close body contact between mother and infant with this type of feeding, it is important to include fathers who may otherwise feel left out. They are also important in the bonding process. Fathers can change nappies or feed expressed milk from the breast, which is put into sterile bottles. They can also assist by putting the infant to the mother's breast and by ensuring the nose is not buried in the breast during feeding.

Mothers must have a good balanced diet in order to make nutritious breast milk, but this is not always economically viable. Also, some substances such as fruit, garlic, spices and alcohol appear in breast milk and may cause colic in the infant. A good fluid intake is also essential, and if mothers feel tired, run-down or are menstruating this may also affect the amount and type of breast milk.

Personal hygiene is important, ensuring the breasts are clean before and after feeding. However, the use of perfumed toiletries should be avoided; the infant uses smell to seek out the breast, so mother's natural pheromones are necessary to encourage feeding. Mothers should wear well-supporting bras and clothes that allow for ease of feeding.

It should be noted that breast feeding is not reliable as a method of contraception.

Bottle feeding with modified milk

Bottle feeding can be done with expressed breast milk, however this method usually means feeding which involves diluting packeted modified baby milks.

Bonding may also occur with bottle feeding and may encourage the whole family's participation, not just mother and infant.

The modified milks are those which have undergone a process of alteration and drying of ordinary cow's milk. This process makes the milk acceptable to an immature gastro–intestinal system. (Refer to Table 6.1.)

Careful preparation of the feed is essential to prevent infection and to ensure correct dilution of solvents and fluid. Incorrect dilution not only gives the infant fewer calories (if solution is too weak), but, if it is too concentrated, can cause the infant to become dehydrated and in electrolyte imbalance.

Some principles to follow when preparing feeds:

— Only make up enough feeds for 24 hours. These should be stored in the fridge.
— Sterile equipment should be used for feed making. Items may be stored in a hypochlorite solution in between feeds.
— Follow the instructions on the packet with regard to dilution of powder to water. Use a level scoop(s) of powder and boiled water.
— Do not add anything to the feed unless directed to do so by the doctor.

Feed times should be relaxed and the infant able to suck easily from the teat. Ensuring that the teat hole is the correct size and that the teat is always full of milk may deter colic. The rooting reflex (p. 136) may assist with bottle feeding, and sucking comes naturally to infants. It is important to pause regularly to rest the infant and to wind him to prevent colic and regurgitation. (This also applies to breast feeding.)

It is easier to see how much fluid the infant is taking when bottle feeding; however accurate estimation may be obtained by a simple calculation. For the first two weeks of postnatal life, infants lose and then regain weight to return to their birth weight. Following that period, 200 gm per week are gained for the next three months. In order to ensure this weight gain, 150 ml milk per expected kg weight must be given over 24 hours, for example:

Calculation of bottle feed requirement for babies up to three months old
Birth weight 3.8 kg
First two weeks lose and regain back to birth weight.
At five weeks the infant should have gained 200 gm per week × 3 (the first 2 weeks are never included).
Therefore 3 × 200 = 600 gm weight gain.
Add this to the birth weight:
3.8 kg + 0.6 kg
= 4.4 kg expected weight at five weeks
To achieve this weight:
4.4 × 150 ml = 660 ml of fluid required in 24 hours,
i.e. 6 feeds per day of 110 ml (4-hourly),
or 5 feeds per day of 132 ml (4-hourly but omitting night feed).
(The night feed is needed for the first couple of months.)

Pre-term infants and those with special needs may require a different calculation of fluid requirements. Infants over three months have a reduced fluid per kilogram expected weight, as calories are also obtained from a weaning diet. An average of 120 g per week is the expected weight gain between three and twelve months.

Table 6.1 Constituents in breast, bottle (modified) and cow's milk (per 100 ml). (From DHSS, 1980)

	BREAST	MODIFIED	COW'S
Calories	70 Kcal	65 Kcal	67 Kcal
Protein	1.2 g (mostly lactalbumin)	1.5 g	3.3 g (mostly casein)
Fat	4.2 g	3.6 g	3.9 g
Carbohydrate	7.1 g (mostly lactose)	7.2 g	4.8 g
Sodium	15 mg (mmol/l)	15 mg	50 mg
Iron	76 mcg	675 mcg	50 mcg

Bottle feeding encourages the whole family to participate in the infant's care. Mother's health will not affect the nutritional requirements of the infant, she can eat any diet and she can feed the infant in any social environment.

Health personnel and facilities

Initial advice about feeding will be given by the midwife. She may visit the mother at home within the first 10 days postnatally. The continuation of care will be taken over by the health visitor who is an important asset to the new mother and infant. She can advise on the practicalities of feeding, teach about feeding, inform about economic benefits, as well as act as a counsellor to the whole family. The health visitor may weigh and assess the infant in the home, or she may see the family at the Health Centre or Clinic.

In some health authorities a Clinical Nurse Specialist: Infant Feeding, may be employed. This person has a joint hospital and community role in infant feeding. The general practitioner is involved in after-care of the mother and in assessing the growth and development of the infant.

Weaning

At around three to four months the infant's calorific requirement changes. This is in line with the more gradual acquisition of weight gain (120 gm per week) and because of other developmental factors. **Weaning** is the gradual introduction of a semi-solid diet and is necessary because of the following factors:

a) Milk cannot provide sufficient calories within the quantity that can be reasonably given to the infant.
b) Iron content in milk is low and this is insufficient to sustain the Hb level of the

infant. The infant is sustained through the first three months of life because of iron transference through the placenta during the last trimester of pregnancy. Iron is stored in the liver. Introduction of substances such as cereals increases iron intake from food.

c) By six months, teeth begin to emerge through the gums, so biting and later chewing is possible.
d) Biting and chewing aid speech development. This becomes obvious where the handicapped child who cannot speak usually has difficulty eating.
e) Taste buds mature and the infant needs to be exposed to differing tastes.
f) Food texture is also important and a weaning diet provides this.

Weaning should be a pleasurable experience for mother and infant, although at first it is not easy and may be quite messy.

Table 6.2 outlines how weaning, and later a more adult diet, may be introduced during the first year of life.

Toddlers and preschool children

The ability to feed oneself is a necessary social skill. Toddlers and preschoolers increase their independence in this field, whilst also absorbing the attitudes of the family to food. There are obviously cultural differences to the progression with independent eating; for instance, in some African countries women breast feed for two years and then suddenly wean the toddler onto a solid diet.

Toddlers and preschoolers can eat most foods, providing salt, sugar, spices and fats are kept under control. By the age of 2½ to 3 years primary dentition (20 teeth) is complete and this assists biting and chewing foods. Taste,

Table 6.2 Changes in nutritional requirements during the first year

AGE	NUTRITIONAL REQUIREMENTS
1–3 months	Breast or bottle (modified) milk feeding.
3–6 months	Around 3–4 months introduce half a diluted teaspoon of cereal at one feed time, e.g. 10 a.m. Cereal is diluted with milk from the allocated quota. This may take one or two weeks to establish. The amount of cereal may be gradually increased. Once one taste is established, a second can be commenced. It is a good idea to try a savoury as infants are not usually as keen as on cereal. A teaspoon of family diet which has been liquidised and diluted with boiled water can be given at one feed time, e.g. 2 p.m. the family food must have been cooked in unsalted water, no table salt added afterwards, and should not be too rich, spicy or fatty. Many parents prefer to buy proprietory tins or packets of savoury food. Towards the end of the first six months, the infant should be eating several different foods, still semi-solid and in gradually increasing quantities. Breast or bottle feeding will continue four-hourly.
6–9 months	During the period six to nine months, the infant is becoming more socially aware and towards the end of this time, may be eating with the family. New recommendations suggest cow's milk should not be introduced until the infant is one year old (DHSS 1988). Fruit juice may be substituted for one or maybe two feeds. This should be of the unsweetened variety, to prevent dental caries. Infants are able to clasp their hands around the bottle and attempt to feed themselves. Others may be using a teacher beaker with handles. Food may become more solid and increase in quantity and tastes. Teeth (incisors) appear around six months and the diet may include fruit or other things to chew on. At this age infants begin to chew anything, so safety must be maintained.
9–12 months	Infants may be placed in a high chair for meal times. By the first birthday, they are likely to be eating at breakfast, lunch and feed times with drinks in between. 1pint (600 ml) milk should still be given daily and this can be cow's milk. The amount of food has increased and one-year-olds often have their own eating plates or bowls and like to attempt to feed themselves with a spoon. Help is very much needed to ensure more food enters the mouth than goes on the floor! Finger feeding is a good resort and is important for manual dexterity and in feeling food texture.

texture and visual attractiveness are issues in encouraging a balanced diet.

Toddlers learn to say 'no' and the beginnings of food fads may emerge. If other members of the family do not like certain foods, the toddler or preschooler may copy them.

Eating utensils should be used with guidance, a fork being gradually introduced.

Checking of weight will help assess the growth and development of the young child. The young child should not be allowed to become too fat, as this may interfere with mobility and may have later consequences on the cardiovascular system.

School children

By the school years children should be able to use a knife, fork and spoon, with reminders about which goes in the mouth. They also have a good idea about what they like and dislike.

Routine is established by school years, so that if the family do not eat breakfast or do not sit down together to eat meals, the school child is likely to follow the same pattern.

At one time, children received school meals, however this system has changed. Some schools offer snacks for lunch and others nothing. This means if children cannot go home for lunch, then they must fend for themselves. Fast food restaurants are often the most accessible and whilst these foods are not totally bad, they should not be eaten all the time.

Children need choices in food; baked beans on brown bread are not bad for children, neither are hamburgers and salad. However, these must be balanced by other food.

School children usually eat well unless ill, tired or stressed. Their social manners need encouraging, such as hand washing, not filling the mouth too full or talking and eating at the same time!

Table 6.3 Changes in nutritional requirements from toddler to adolescent (Whaley & Wong 1979)

DAILY REQUIREMENTS	TODDLER 1–3 YEARS	PRESCHOOLER 4–6 YEARS	SCHOOLCHILD 7–10 YEARS	ADOLESCENT 11–18 YEARS	
Calories	1300 Kcal	1800 Kcal	2400 Kcal	2800 to 3000 Kcal	2400 to 3000 Kcal
Protein	23 g	30 g	36 g	44–54 g	44–48 g
Fats	These form part of the energy requirements of children, but need to be carefully regulated.				
Iron	15 mg	10 mg	10 mg	18 mg	18 mg
Calcium	800 mg	800 mg	800 mg	1200 mg	1200 mg
Vitamin D	400 iu	400 iu	400 iu	400 iu	400 iu

Adolescence

By adolescence, patterns of eating and likes and dislikes are firmly established. There is an increased demand for calories associated with the growth surge of puberty. Girls may appear chubby during this time and boys awkward and disproportionate in body and limbs.

The adolescent is very aware of his body image and associates diet with this. For instance, acne, which is due to pubertal hormonal changes, may be associated with too much fat in the diet. Adolescent girls may try

Table 6.4 Average weights from infancy to adolescence

GIRLS		BOYS	
AGE	WEIGHT (kg)	AGE	WEIGHT (kg)
Birth	3.4	Birth	3.4
1	9.6	1	10.3
3	14.4	3	14.6
5	18.3	5	18.3
7	23.6	7	24.5
9	28.9	9	29.9
11–14	44.0	11–14	44.0
15–18	54.0	15–18	60.0

to diet, either because their friends are slimmer or they are called names, like 'fatty', or because they can't wear the clothes they would like; there is a danger at this stage of anorexia nervosa. Whilst this condition is not common, adolescent girls are particularly at risk.

Adolescent boys may have ravenous appetities and always be hungry. Food is also associated with a good body physique, which in turn is part of physical and sexual attractiveness.

Developmental aspects

Fluid balance in infants and older children

In infancy the total body water is nearly 80% of the infant's body weight. Body water is distributed between intra- and extracellular compartments, with 35% of body weight being in the intracellular compartments and 45% extracellularly.

This difference from adult fluid balance changes rapidly in the first ten days of the neonatal period and adult distribution of fluid is reached by two years of age. In the first year, for instance, the extracellular fluid percentage decreases from 45% to 27%, with a relative increase in the intracellular fluid compartment. The principal electrolytes in the extracellular fluid are sodium (Na^+) and chloride (Cl^-), and because of the fluid available outside the cells, loss of fluid also means loss of these electrolytes.

The changes in the first ten days are due mainly to insensible loss. Only half the total body water is intracellular by the first birthday, compared with the adult who has two-thirds intracellularly. The infant's fluid balance is easily disturbed and any fluid loss or gain is relatively greater in magnitude and effect than in adults. If this is considered in relation to the facts that (a) infants cannot physically regulate fluid intake and output for themselves, (b) their basal metabolic rate (BMR) is three times that of adults, (c) their body surface to weight ratio is greater than in adults, which increases the insensible loss area, and (d) their kidneys cannot concentrate or conserve water, then it becomes apparent that fluid regulation is of crucial importance. The changes which occur to give the adult water distribution are due to muscle growth, an increase in cell size (especially nerve cells) and a general increase in all organs.

The gastro–intestinal tract

The physiological and biochemical functions of the gastro–intestinal tract are established at birth, but digestive processes do not function maturely until three months of age.

The infant can suck and swallow by an automatic reflex action which becomes co-ordinated and controlled when the nervous system matures. Weaning at three months takes advantage of this fact. Chewing is aided by dental development. The infant produces little saliva and any enzymes present do not have time to act on quickly-swallowed milk.

The stomach is small and round, elongating by two years old. In infancy digestive enzymes are present, but do not work effectively until the pH is determined. Gastric acidity is low during this time and rennin, an enzyme, is secreted to act on casein in milk to form curds.

Secretions into the gastro–intestinal tract are proportionately greater than in adults, because of the relative size of this system in infants. There is an increased predisposition to dehydration partly for this reason, and partly because the tract is immunologically immature and at risk of infection and inflammation (diarrhoea).

Peristalsis is rapid and food passes quickly through the tract. (Further consideration of the lower GI tract will be found in Chapter 7, Elimination and personal cleansing and dressing.)

The liver is not able to conjugate bilirubin and effectively secrete bile until after the first two weeks of life, consequently young infants often have a physiological jaundice, which disappears gradually in the first one or two weeks and is improved by a good fluid intake.

Dentition – primary

From approximately six months to two and a half years primary deciduous dentition takes place. The order in which teeth appear is given in Table 6.5.

Dental hygiene is considered in Chapter 7, Eliminating, personal cleansing and dressing. Tooth development assists not only with eating, but also with speech.

Dentition – secondary

Secondary teeth are the permanent set which start to erupt in school children and continue into early adulthood. If wisdom teeth are present, the total numbers 32. From the age of six or seven years, the school child loses four

Table 6.5 Primary dentition

APPROXIMATE AGE	TEETH
6–7 months	2 lower central incisors
9 months	2 upper central incisors
	2 upper lateral incisors
1 year	2 lower lateral incisors
14 months	4 first molars
18 months	4 canines
2–2½ years	4 second molars
Total 20 teeth	

deciduous teeth per year and gradually replaces these by permanent teeth, including four additional molars, until early adolescence. The most obvious loss is that of the central incisors around six to eight years, causing a 'gappy' smile.

Growth and development

Although eating and drinking are closely tied up with the accepted growth and development norms of childhood, they will be considered more fully in Chapter 8, Mobilising, working, playing and sleeping.

CHECK LIST

Assessment of the child's eating and drinking

1 Ask parents about the child's eating and drinking routine. How much food? how often? and of what type? are important considerations. Are there any likes or dislikes?
2 Were there any feeding difficulties in infancy or any problems with weaning?
3 Was weight gain satisfactory? Weigh the child.
4 *Current status of the child*
   — Vomiting: how much, how often, colour, consistency
   — Diarrhoea: how much, how often, colour, consistency
   — Any pain or distension, e.g. abdominal, causing pain
   — Weight loss
   — Weight gain (check for oedema)
   — Hydration

Warnings of dehydration may include: altered or elevated pulse and respiratory rate; blood pressure may be difficult to record; colour may be poor; if fever is present, then temperature will be elevated.

Features associated with dehydration in the older child may be similar, except of course,

Fig. 6.1 Features associated with dehydration in the infant

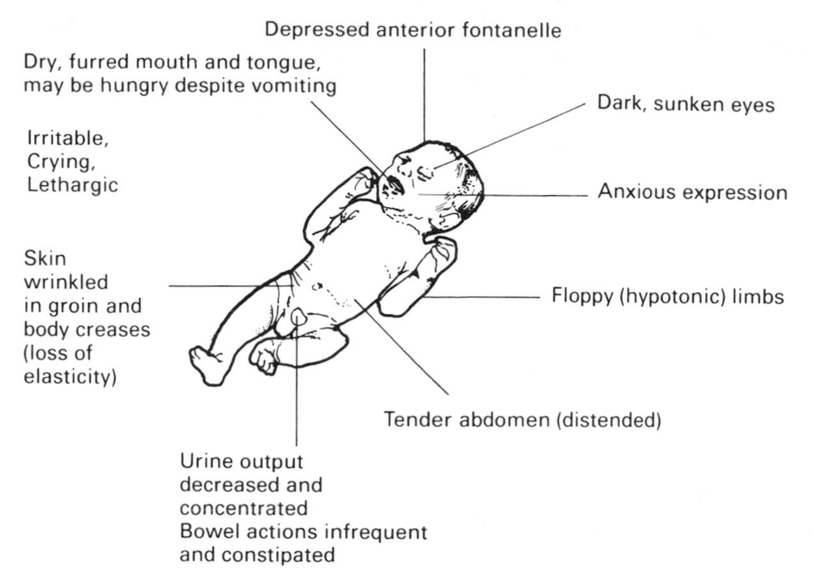

the fontanelle will be fused by 18 months. The features may be less severe, however children should not be left in a state where fluid loss and electrolyte imbalance may endanger health. Likewise, weight gain associated with oedema should receive immediate attention.

CARE PLAN

An infant with pyloric stenosis

Nikki Alexander was the first-born boy of Jeffrey and Jane. He was born without difficulty, cried lustily and fed hungrily for the first few weeks of life. When Nikki reached six weeks of age, he suddenly started to vomit and this vomiting was projectile in nature.

Nikki was admitted to the ward as an emergency, as Jane had taken him to the GP after he had vomited twice. Suspecting an obstruction to the upper gastro–intestinal tract, the GP arranged for Nikki to be admitted straightaway. On admission Nikki had vomited three times, was fractious, crying and chewing his fist hungrily. Jane also mentioned that he had passed one small, hard, greenish stool that morning. Jane was obviously very worried and guilty about the state of Nikki and needed explanation and reassurance before she was able to settle in the cubicle with her infant. Following a medical history, examination and test feed, the doctor made a provisional diagnosis of pyloric stenosis.

Pyloric stenosis (congenital hypertrophic pyloric stenosis) This disorder is a congenital obstruction of the pyloric sphincter. The pyloric muscle hypertrophies and thickens and presses inwards on the lumen of the pylorus, so causing obstruction to the outflow of contents from the stomach. The stomach dilates, gastric emptying is delayed and irritation may cause gastric bleeding. The disorder does not usually become apparent until a few weeks after birth and is commoner in males than females (6:1). It is also more common in white Caucasian infants than in infants of West Indian origin.

ADMISSION TO HOSPITAL

A nursing and medical history was taken from Jane about Nikki. This followed the check list on page 110. Nikki was found to be dehydrated, vomiting projectily with small flecks of blood present in the vomit. His weight, which was 3.4 kg at birth, was now 3.8 kg (at six weeks, 4.2 kg would be the expected weight).

On palpation of the abdomen, a small olive-shaped 'tumour' was felt and later observed when a test feed was given to Nikki. Peristaltic waves going from left to right across the epigastrium were also seen.

Care plan for Nikki during the acute phase

Correction of dehydration

Because Nikki was so obviously dehydrated, immediate medical intervention was necessary. A vein in the scalp was exposed after shaving away some hair (Nikki's mum needed much reassurance about this) and a cannula inserted and carefully secured in position. (In young infants veins in the scalp are nearer the surface than those in small, mobile limbs, and it may be less likely that the infant can knock the cannula out of place.) Alkalosis is most likely with vomiting, due to the loss of HCl, potassium and chlorides. Other blood tests will show increased haematocrit and haemoglobin because of reduced fluid volume.

Care of an intravenous infusion

1 Ensure the cannula is secured in position, and check the infusion site regularly.
2 Ensure the giving set tubing cannot become entangled round the infant, or become kinked or compressed. Ensure no air bubbles or blood in the tubing.
3 It may be necessary to put mittens on an infant to stop tiny fingers pulling out the cannula.
4 Ensure correct fluid is infused and check the rate frequently. A burette and an infusion pump are often used to regulate the giving of small quantities of fluids to infants. The pump needs checking regularly to ensure correct functioning.
5 Record input and output hourly on a fluid balance chart.
6 Check for signs of overloading, such as respiratory difficulties or raised pulse rate, every half hour.

Care plan for Nikki during the rehydration phase and pre-operatively

PROBLEM 1

Problem
Vomiting leading to dehydration and (p) altered level of consciousness.
(p) apnoea and altered respiratory status.

Aims of nursing care
Maintain a patent airway.
Alleviate vomiting, ensure rehydration schedule achieved.

NURSING CARE

Place Nikki in a cot with the head end raised and with him lying propped on his side, to maintain a patent airway.

Observe Nikki's response to communication to ascertain conscious level.

Assist doctor with commencing an intravenous infusion and maintain this (see p. 113). Record half-hourly pulse and respiratory rate, hourly temperature and fluid recordings. Test vomit, urine and stools for blood.

Under supervision (or by observation) insert a naso-gastric tube to aspirate gastric contents. Securely tape the tube in position and aspirate hourly and whenever retching occurs, otherwise allow tube to drain freely. Record aspirate and test for blood. Observe general state of hydration. Encourage Jane to clean Nikki's mouth with cotton wool or cotton buds every half hour to an hour. Nikki should be given nothing by mouth.

EVALUATION

Nikki's state of hydration, vital signs, and blood electrolytes will indicate if rehydration is successful.

PROBLEM 2

Problem
(p) for infection, due to immature immune system and debilitated physical state.

Aim of nursing care
Prevent infection.

NURSING CARE

Nurse Nikki in a protective isolation cubicle with all his own equipment. Ensure correct handwashing before contact and wear appropriate gowns and aprons. (Refer to Chapter 2, Maintaining a safe environment.)

Nikki may also get rest and sleep by being placed in a quiet environment. This also allows for parents to be resident. Jane had a bed beside Nikki's cot which encouraged her to remain in contact with Nikki and all his care and treatment.

EVALUATION

No infection should be acquired whilst in hospital. Nikki's vital signs may indicate an infection; chest infection and post-operative wound infection are the most likely.

PROBLEM 3

Problem	*Aims of nursing care*
Anxiety of Jane and Jeffrey because of Nikki's emergency admission, poor health and planned surgery. Nikki is fractious and irritable.	Minimise anxiety by involvement in care and frequent informative explanation about Nikki. Comfort, pacify and distract.

NURSING CARE

Explain to Jane (and later to Jeffrey when present) the nursing care associated with dehydration and the importance of frequent observations. Ensure the medical staff explain pyloric stenosis, all investigations and treatment and the need for surgery. The doctor should obtain consent to operation from the parents.

Encourage Jane to handle and comfort Nikki. Parents are likely to feel guilty and unable to do anything whilst Nikki has an infusion and naso-gastric tube. However, cuddling, touching, general and oral hygiene and nappy changing can all be done by the parents. Jane may like to put brightly coloured mobiles and toys on the bed. Small, safe and cuddly toys are also suitable and may distract Nikki from feeling hungry.

EVALUATION

Anxiety of Nikki's parents and Nikki's fractiousness will not resolve until surgery has been performed.

Pyloromyotomy (Ramstedt's operation) is division of the pyloric muscle to allow protrusion of the muscle sphincter away from the lumen.
Surgery is not performed until the infant is in fluid and electrolyte balance. This may cause a delay of operation for 24 to 48 hours.
It may be necessary for the infant to have several gastric washouts with isotonic (normal) saline, pre-operatively. The washouts clear the stomach of any milk curds and stale blood. Abdominal X-rays or ultrasound and barium meals are other investigations sometimes ordered.

Nikki's pre-operative and post-operative care

(Refer to Chapter 2, Maintaining a safe environment.)

Special aspects of post-operative care following a pyloromyotomy

Dependent on the surgeon's instructions, feeding orally may commence 2–6 hours after surgery. Glucose water (or an electrolyte mixture) is given first and gradually the infant is regraded back on to full-strength milk. Breast-fed babies are able to suckle again, four hours post-operatively. The intravenous infusion is likely to be maintained until feeding is established.

If vomiting occurs, then the feeding regime reverts back to the previous stage. 'Winding' during feeding is important and the infant's head should be elevated after the feed.

SUBSEQUENT CARE AND PARENTAL EDUCATION

Nikki may be discharged home when the following criteria have been met:

1 Full strength milk feeds are tolerated
2 No vomiting
3 No clinical signs of dehydration (including electrolyte balance)
4 Gaining weight
5 Wound is healing
6 Temperature is not elevated
7 Parents feel able to cope at home

Jane would be advised to let her health visitor know that she is at home with Nikki. The GP will receive a letter from the hospital and the district nurse would be contacted to visit and remove Nikki's sutures around the fifth or sixth post-operative day. Jane should know how to care for the wound, keeping it clean and free of urine and faeces. Nikki may demand more frequent attention until he settles at home and Jane may be worried about leaving him in case he vomits. She should be reassured that recurrence is unlikely and that any subsequent children won't necessarily be affected.

A follow-up hospital appointment will be given and the ward telephone number in case Jane needs advice.

EXERCISE

An adolescent girl admitted for treatment of obesity

Obesity is defined as 'an increase in the body weight resulting from an excessive accumulation of fat, or simply the state of being too fat' (Whaley & Wong 1983).

Mary Smithers, 15 years old, weighed 57 kg and despite attempts by her mother to encourage Mary to diet, she continued to gain rather than lose weight. Mary had passed through puberty at the age of 13, when she also started menstruating. Since that time she had developed a large appetite and seemed unable to control this, despite being depressed with her physical appearance. Her friends constantly teased Mary about her size.

On admission to hospital Mary waddled into the ward looking very fed up and was uncommunicative. It was noticed that Mrs Smithers also had a weight problem.

1 Causes of obesity

Using the following headings, suggest at least one cause of obesity for each:

a) Age-related (i.e. adolescence)
b) Familial
c) Endocrine (there are at least two different target organs)
d) Inheritance and genetic
e) Psychosocial

2 Identifying Mary's problems

Using the introductory background material given about Mary Smithers, identify the problems which would need to be included in her plan of care.

a) *Identified problems prioritised*
b) *Suggest ways in which Mary's problems may be overcome using nursing care and prescribed treatment*
c) *How may Mary be educated about controlling her weight when she is discharged from hospital?*

Information to assist with the exercises

(i) The *Activities of Living Framework* (Roper *et al.* 1985) may serve as a basis for establishing a normal routine and in identification of problems (actual and potential)
(ii) *Adolescence* and changes related to this age must be borne in mind at all times. (Chapters 3, 6, 7 and 8 may be useful for this)
(iii) Consider the *practical aspects* of encouraging a child to eat, especially an adolescent who is nearly independent

from her family and can make choices and decisions

(iv) Losing weight requires *motivation*

(v) Obesity results from a calorific intake which exceeds expenditure.

REFERENCES

DHSS. 1988. *Present Day Practice in Infant Feeding.* Report of a working party of the panel on child nutrition. Committee on Medical Aspects of Food Policy. Report on Health and Social Subjects No. 32 (Chairman T. E. Oppe). HMSO, London.

ROPER, N., LOGAN, W. & TIERNEY, A. J. 1985. *The Elements of Nursing,* 2nd Edn. Churchill Livingstone, London.

WHALEY, L. F. & WONG, D. L. 1983. *Nursing Care of Infants and Sick Children,* 2nd Edn. Mosby, St Louis.

FURTHER READING

FRANCIS, D. 1986. *Nutrition for Children.* Blackwell Scientific Press, Oxford.

MCLAREN, D. S. & BURMAN, D. (Eds) 1982. *Textbook of Paediatric Nutrition,* 2nd Edn. Churchill Livingstone, Edinburgh.

TAYLOR, T. G. 1982. *Nutrition and Health.* Studies in Biology, No 141. Edward Arnold, London.

7 Eliminating, personal cleansing and dressing

The development of autonomy is linked with mastering many physical and social skills. Elimination, cleansing and dressing are considered in this chapter. By the time the child reaches school age he is usually able to care for these activities of living, however when placed in a new or stressful environment (e.g. school) he may show signs of regression until he feels comfortable and in control of the situation.

The care plan used to illustrate this chapter is in the form of an exercise which needs completion by the reader. The child is a six-year-old admitted to hospital with constipation and soiling. He is discovered also to have head lice.

Health promotion and education

Infants

Elimination

The infant urinates 90 ml per day at birth with an output of 450–600 ml in 24 hours at one year. There is no control over micturition, due to immaturity of the nervous system and lack of learned behaviour. Bowels are opened after every feed during the first few months of life. Faeces change character and consistency during the first year:

— **Meconium** is the sticky black tarry substance passed for the first days after birth. It consists of cast-off epithelial cells, digestive tract secretions (mucus) and residue from the swallowed amniotic fluid.

- **A changing stool** is produced when milk feeds become established at the end of the first week and the consistency is meconium and pale curds.
- **Breast-fed** babies produce more frequent, pale yellow and semi-soft stools, these often contain curds and are more acidic than the stools of bottle-fed babies.
- **Bottle-fed** babies on modified milks tend to have darker yellow and more formed stools.
- When **weaning** is established stools become more bulky, darker in colour and by the end of the first year are passed once or twice a day.

Infants should be washed, dried and the nappy changed after every urination and defaecation. Ammonia left on the skin is an irritant and can cause skin breakdown and nappy rash. Barrier creams may be applied.

Cleansing

Bathing once a day is usually sufficient for the infant, with 'top and tail' washes in between. Parents can also inspect the body from head to toe.

Hair and scalp Wash with baby soap or shampoo. Inspect for a brown scurf called 'cradle cap' (oil-based compounds will loosen this; these can then be washed off). Gently feel the anterior fontanelle for location and closure (and as an indicator of hydration). Brush hair with a baby brush.

Eyes Tears are not secreted until the tear ducts are fully formed. Gentle cleansing with sterile water can minimise infection.

Ears Clear with cotton wool to remove wax, vomit, etc. Cotton buds may penetrate too far along the straight, short, external auditory canal.

Nose (see also Chapter 4, Breathing) Clear with cotton wool. Milia (milk spots) may appear on the nose and should be left to disappear in their own time, being blocked sebaceous glands.

Mouth This should be clear and moist and show no evidence of *Candida* (an oral infection). After six months teeth may be visible and towards the end of the first year a soft toothbrush may be used.

Body and limbs Wash and dry all skin surfaces, particularly in skin creases and the umbilicus.

Nails These are soft and peel off at first. Later, cutting should be done to prevent scratching.

Genitalia Ensure no excoriation. Clean with soap and water. In boys the testes should be in the scrotum. In young female infants the labia may look swollen, but this is quite normal.

Dressing

Infants need layers of clothes, preferably cotton and non-irritant. Bonnets, bootees and mittens are necessary to keep the extremities warm.

Clothes should allow for movement and not restrict growth (e.g. feet in babygrows). The socialisation process may be enhanced by particular clothes and colours dependent on gender.

Toddlers and preschool children

Elimination

Toilet training is an age-old 'chestnut' in child development. The combination of physical and psychological 'letting go' may be acquired for defaecation before control of urination at two to three years in the daytime. Nighttime urine control may be finally acquired by four to five years. Withholding fluids in the evening may be a useful technique. Most schools like children to be toilet trained before commencing their education.

Toilet training may be helped by employing the following suggestions:

1 A potty placed next to the 'adult' lavatory. Use of this may be encouraged by role modelling from older siblings or parents.
2 A small seat which can fix on to the standard toilet seat. Children are frightened of slipping through the hole, so this may prevent anxiety.
3 Steps (portable) leading up to the toilet.
4 No locks on the bathroom or toilet doors.

5 Reward good and dry behaviour and do not scold when accidents occur.

Children should be shown how to wipe themselves after using the toilet and encouraged to wash and dry their hands.

Personal cleansing

Young children like to attempt to care for themselves and a degree of experimentation is important for the toddler and preschooler. However, safety is still the most important consideration, especially where hot water is being used. Encourage young children to learn to run cold water into a bath before adding hot water and always stay with them during the bath, as youngsters can drown in just one inch of water. Children of this age do not always wash themselves as thoroughly as adults would like, so assistance is needed.

Dental hygiene, started in late infancy, must be continued with regular and correct brushing of teeth and visits to the dentist.

Dressing

Toddlers and preschool children learn to dress themselves quite rapidly. By three years old, the child dresses by himself almost completely. The toddler however can still be indiscriminate in showing off new clothes, particularly underwear. He can take off gloves, socks and shoes, unzip clothes and make a good attempt at putting arms and legs into garments – sometimes back to front! The preschooler can dress, doing up front buttons and sides of clothes and puts on socks and shoes.

Schoolchildren and adolescents

Elimination

By school age, the child should be toilet trained, however accidents can still occur, where facilities are inadequate or when the child is put in a stressed environment. The first weeks at school or admission to hospital may cause a degree of regression in elimination, however this should resolve. Privacy and hygiene remain important when eliminating.

Personal cleansing

By five years, the child is virtually self-caring; but supervision should still be given with baths. Children are so busy learning that washing is considered an interruption to their activities and is carried out quickly and without attention to detail. Nails, knees and ears are just some parts of the body which can get overlooked!

Cleaning teeth should be continued, as well as dental visits, remembering that from around the age of six or seven years, children will begin to lose their primary teeth and replace them with permanent teeth.

Adolescents have their own attitude to personal cleanliness, either being over-zealous, or not bothering. Acne can appear on the face and hair grows under arms, where perspiration carries an odour. Boys begin to shave or grow a stubble. Menstrual hygiene is important for girls who have reached the menarche.

Dressing

School children can dress themselves completely, needing help initially with back buttons, ties and shoe laces. They begin to make choices in what to wear, girls often liking pretty clothes. Bows, ribbons and jewellery may begin to be worn. Children get engrossed in what they are doing and forget to dress appropriately, for instance in cold weather, when mittens or gloves and hats are needed, so checking the child's dress should continue. Adolescents experiment with clothes, appearing to lack coordination of colour, style and so on. This is part of establishing their own image and together with clothes, hairstyles, makeup and jewellery form part of this image. Fashion has to be followed implicity and usually relates to an idol or role model. Dressing an adolescent who is not earning can become costly, because fashions change from season to season.

Developmental aspects

1 The genito–urinary system

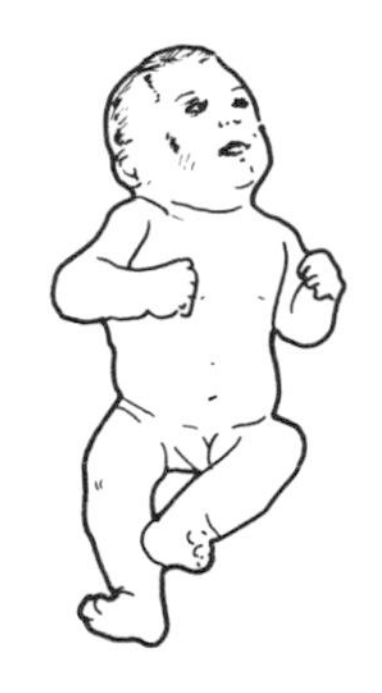

Urine accumulates in the bladder, proprioceptors within the muscle tissues are activated by the stretching of the walls. Impulses sent by visceral afferents
↓
Spinal cord via the autonomic nervous system
↓
Causes smooth muscle to contract the bladder wall
↓
Urine is expelled

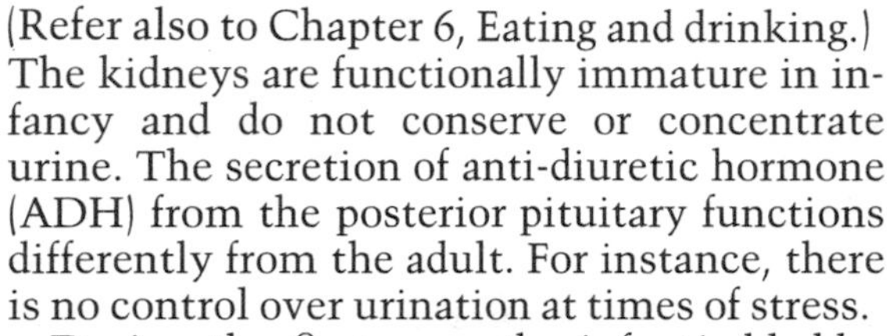

(Refer also to Chapter 6, Eating and drinking.) The kidneys are functionally immature in infancy and do not conserve or concentrate urine. The secretion of anti-diuretic hormone (ADH) from the posterior pituitary functions differently from the adult. For instance, there is no control over urination at times of stress.

During the first year, the infant's bladder capacity increases considerably. By 14–18 months, the child is able to retain urine for up to two hours or more. The child needs to develop awareness of the sensation to urinate and to be able to communicate this to parents.

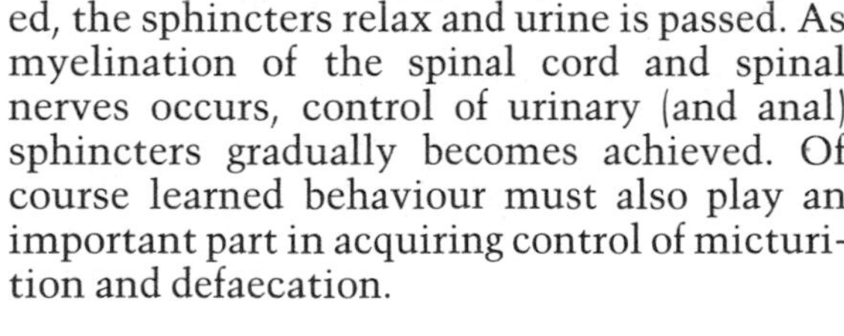

At first urination occurs due to a spinal reflex. When the bladder receptors are stretched, the sphincters relax and urine is passed. As myelination of the spinal cord and spinal nerves occurs, control of urinary (and anal) sphincters gradually becomes achieved. Of course learned behaviour must also play an important part in acquiring control of micturition and defaecation.

2 The gastro–intestinal tract

(Refer also to Chapter 6, Eating and drinking.) The bowel in infants is short in length and therefore foods such as peas, carrots, corn and raisins may pass through without being digested. Although the bowel is short, the gastro–intestinal tract is proportionately larger in infants than in adults and this predisposes to a greater water loss. Secretions in the tract are also greater.

Myelination of nerves which control defaecation occurs at the same time as those affecting the genito–urinary system.

Initially, when the infant's rectum is stimulated by faeces, the anal sphincters open and the bowels are emptied. As peristalsis is rapid and bowel length short, it is quite normal for infants to defaecate after every feed. As the nervous system matures, appropriate social behaviour is learned and diet becomes more solid, so the number and type of faeces change. The time and place for defaecation also becomes under the control of the child.

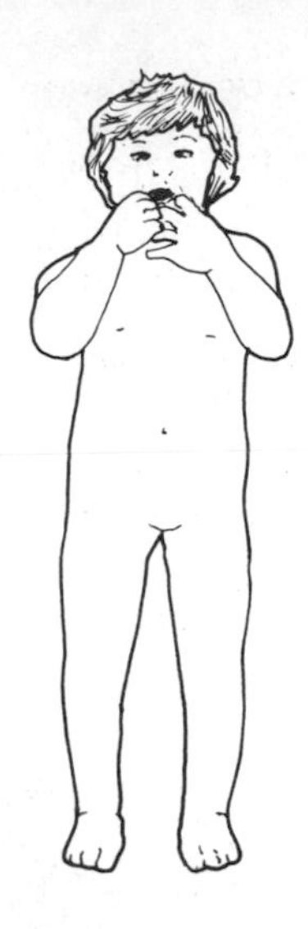

Urine is formed and accumulates in the bladder in the same way as in infants. However, the toddler learns to understand the sensation of a full bladder. Learning when to void urine is assisted by the development of a social awareness, maturation of the nervous system and learning when to 'hold on' or 'let go' (sphincter control).

3 The integumentary system

(Refer also to Chapter 5, Maintaining body temperature.)
The ratio of the infant's surface area to body weight is greater than in the adult, therefore greater insensible loss of fluid can occur. Also the basal metabolic rate being higher, subsequent loss of heat may be greater.

The binding together of the skin's layers, the dermis and epidermis, occurs during infancy and this assists with protection against infection. Small amounts of sweat begin to be produced and also sebum which protects and nourishes the skin. Initially infants are predisposed to dry skin (e.g. cradle cap) and to skin infections and excoriation such as nappy rash.

CHECK LIST

Assessment of the child's elimination, personal cleansing and dressing

1 Is the child toilet trained or wearing nappies? (It is important not to be judgemental about toilet training, as it is extremely individual to each family.)

2 If the child is toilet trained, when did this commence and are any special pieces of equipment used (e.g. steps to reach toilet)? How often does the child use the toilet?
3 If difficulties have arisen, such as enuresis, encopresis or constipation, do parents have any ideas what might have precipitated the onset?
4 Is the child in pain? Does he look worried or anxious?
5 Do the parents have a routine for personal cleansing and dressing?
6 What is the state of the child's skin; are there any rashes or marks? Is the skin healthy-looking and a good colour?
7 How much can the child care for himself?
8 Is the child going to wear his own clothes and are there any special items of clothing?

EXERCISE

A six-year-old boy admitted with constipation, soiling and head lice

Background information

Tommy Tipping lived on the edge of a large town with his mother and seven-year-old sister, Theresa. He attended a school near home and had been toilet trained before commencing school at five years old. Unfortunately, Tommy's father had run off with a new girlfriend when Tommy had just had his fifth birthday. Although he had seen his father once or twice since, Tommy found it difficult to understand why his dad no longer lived at home. Tommy's mum had been devastated when this happened and at first coped with the family by being very authoritarian. Latterly, however, she appeared not to care about herself or the family and Theresa had become very naughty and constantly misbehaved.

The school teacher noticed that Tommy began to smell, and with very careful observation and talking to Tommy, she discovered that he frequently soiled his pants and rarely went to the toilet 'properly'. The school medical team were involved and Tommy's mother was contacted, to try and help resolve the situation. However, by the age of six, Tommy was so constipated that he needed to be admitted to the paediatric ward, both to clear his constipation and for investigations.

Admission to the paediatric ward

Tommy is admitted to the ward, with his mother and Theresa, but mum does not wish to be resident. The bed area selected for Tommy is with other school children, but in the corner of the ward to provide privacy. The whole family are made to feel welcome and shown around the ward, including bathrooms, toilets, play area and parents' kitchen and rest room.

As part of the admission assessment the nurse examines Tommy's head and discovers head lice.

Check the following before answering the questions below:
a) Knowledge of a normal 6-year-old child's development, especially in relation to elimination.
b) Remind yourself of the 12 Activities of Living and using a chart (see Fig. 1.1, p. 8), identify where Tommy is along each continuum.
c) Using the 12 Activities of Living (or a guidelines sheet used in your Health Authority) establish Tommy's normal routine and any actual or (p) potential problems. Chapters 2, 3, 6 and 8 may assist you.

1 Outline the psychosocial factors which may have contributed to Tommy's present admission to hospital.

2 What physical abnormalities may have caused Tommy's constipation and soiling? State the relevant investigations which might be performed, to assist with the diagnosis.

3 a) Establish a priority order for the problems listed in Fig. 7.2, and add any other problems you considered should be included.

Fig. 7.2 Tommy Tipping may present with the problems listed below

Problems	Goals	Action	Evaluation
(Not in priority order, see Question 3a) - Constipation and soiling - Decreased ability to maintain a safe environment due to new surroundings - Head lice and nits - Anxiety due to new environment and leaving home and family - (p) Inadequate, low-fibre diet, predisposing to constipation - (p) Anxiety about missing school and friends - (p) Fear and anxiety about treatment and care which involves private (sexual) body parts			

b) Complete the chart given in Fig. 7.2 (under supervision) by stating goals, action and evaluation.

4 What initial treatment should be given for Tommy's head lice and nits (include the names and actions of relevant lotions)? What education should be given to Tommy's mum to prevent recurrence of head lice?

5 What personnel and support systems exist to help Tommy's mum at this time of personal stress? What are your feelings about Tommy's mother and are they likely to affect your ability to support her?

REFERENCE

ROBERTS, C. 1987. A lousy life. *Community Outlook*, (August), 16–19.

8 Mobilising, working, playing and sleeping

The child's ability to mobilise depends on his developmental stage and this in turn relates to his physical stature. From birth to adolescence the development in mobility cannot be surpassed at any other stage of life. Play is of paramount importance to a child's development; how he plays depends on his degree of mobility and play is also a child's work. Play links the transition for the child from home to school, where work (education) is formalised and a legal requirement from 5–16 years. Schooling is extremely important and most children do not like to miss it. Children need sufficient rest and sleep in order to have the energy to play and the concentration to work.

This chapter considers all these aspects and uses a handicapped child as the care plan illustration of a child with gross mobility problems, but also shows how these affect many other activities of living.

Health promotion and education

The infant will be assessed at birth for physical development. This includes height, weight and head circumference and use of the Apgar Scale. The midwife or doctor uses an Apgar score to ascertain heart rate, respiratory effort, colour, reflex irritability and muscle tone. Each infant is given a score out of ten, this assessment being made at one, five and ten minutes. Most infants score between 7 and 10 on the Apgar Scale. Frequent observation of development is necessary in the first years of life. For the first ten days, the midwife will visit and assess the infant as well as being an adviser to parents. From 10 days up until five years, the health visitor has a key role. She or the GP in the Health Clinic will assess development in all fields; fine motor, gross motor, sight and hearing at approximately six weeks, seven months, 15 months, 2½ and 4½ years. Often these developmental assessments will coincide with clinic visits for immunisation. The basis of most assessments comes from a system known as *The Denver Developmental Screening Test* (Frankenburg & Dodds 1969).

The infant and then the child's development (height, weight and head circumference) will be plotted along a centile chart, to ascertain if he is within the normal range of development for his age.

How the infant develops is not only determined by his physical attributes or characteristics with which he was born (nature) but also the environment in which he grows up (nurture). Even a severely handicapped child, if nurtured carefully, can show small improvements in physical and mental development.

Once the child goes to school and up until the end of adolescence, the school medical team take over the regular developmental assessments. Although the assessments are usually performed by the doctor, the school nurse may provide important information about the child which may affect development, by virtue of the fact that she may be with the children more frequently. Referrals to paediatricians can be made if any abnormalities are found at assessment.

Developmental aspects

The direction of growth occurs in several ways. Firstly the infant grows and develops **cephalocaudally** (head to toe) and secondly **proximodistally** (development of the limbs from near to the body, out to fingers and toes).

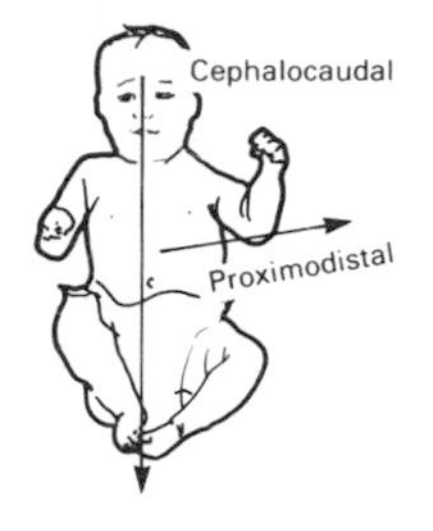

The child's physical proportions alter rapidly between infancy and adolescence. The infant's head to body ratio is approximately 1:3 or 1:4 and there is no head control, no curves in the spine and reactions to the environment are primitive, because of an immature nervous system. During the toddler, preschool and school years the child lengthens and becomes more proportionate in head, body and limb ratio. Curves in the spine appear first at the cervical region with head control and secondly in the lumbar spine with crawling and walking. Maturation of the nervous system suppresses primitive movements and movement and behaviour become learned and purposeful. By adolescence, the body has undergone a pubertal growth spurt, maturation of internal organs and sexual development. Puberty is brought about by changes in the levels of sexual hormones. Until the pubertal period subsides, adolescents may be awkward in movement.

Neonatal reflexes

During the neonatal period (28 days) strong primitive reflexes can be noted and elicited from the neonate. The reflexes are reactions to stimuli in the environment and primitive because they appear to serve no purpose and do not relate to purposeful behaviour. As the nervous system matures, with development of the brain, myelination of nerves and the neonate's exposure to life, so these reflexes gradually fade. Most have disappeared by three months of age. The most common reflexes are listed below; there are in all more than 30 which can be sought.

1 **Moro reflex** Sometimes called a startle reflex. Elicited by unbalancing the head or

Fig. 8.1 Changes in height and weight from 0–15 years in girls and boys

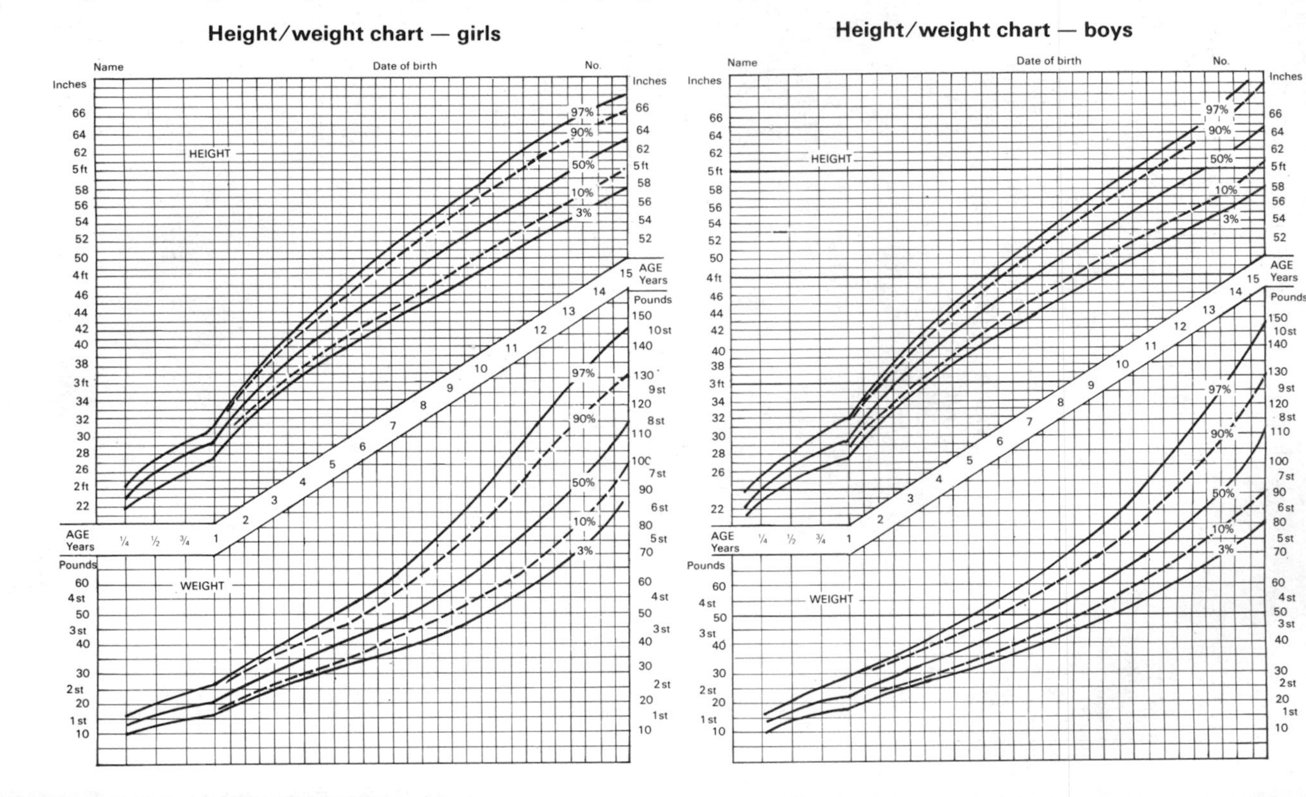

Fig. 8.2 The changing proportion of head, body and limbs from birth to adulthood

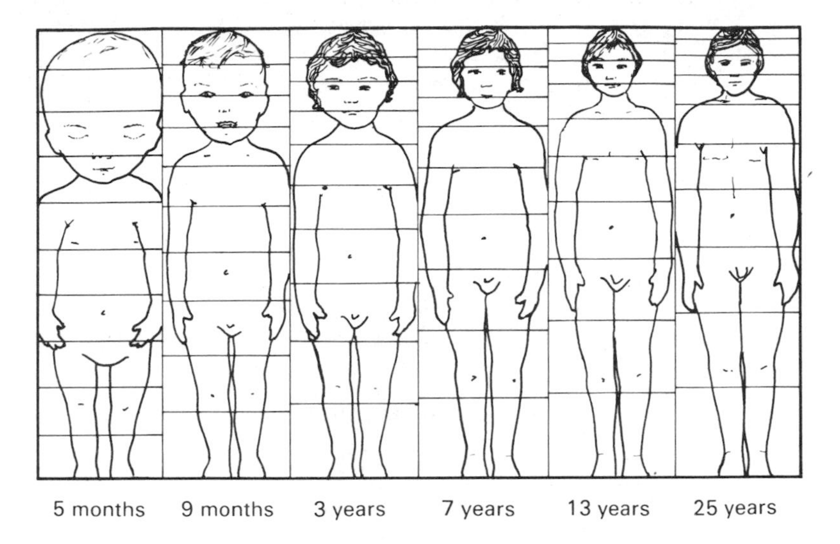

jarring of the cot. The infant throws out his arms and opens his hands in a movement associated with balance. He then draws his arms back into his body and regrasps his fingers. Fades by six weeks. Disappears by three months.

2 **Tonic neck reflex** If the head is turned from one side to the other, the arm and leg on the side that the head is turned extend, and the opposite arm and leg flex. If the head is turned in the other direction, the limbs also alter. This is probably a safety and balance reflex. Fades and disappears by three to four months.

3 **Grasp reflex** If a finger is placed in the ulnar side of the infant's palm, he will grasp tightly. It is possible that he can be lifted up by this grasp if two hands are held. It can be uncomfortable and potentially unsafe to do this unless necessary. Fades and lessens by three months, replaced by voluntary grasp.

4 **Walking/stepping/placing reflex** If the infant's feet are placed on a firm surface, he will lift each foot alternately as if walking. Proper walking will not commence until the end of the first year or subsequently. Fades and disappears at three to four weeks.

5 **Rooting reflex** Touching the cheek adjacent to the mouth encourages the infant to seek the source of touch in order to suck it. The touching is associated with the nipple which the infant must seek in order to feed. It is a useful reflex for breast and bottle feeding. Fades and disappears at three to four months but can persist until twelve months.

Changes to the cranium

Head circumference, which is normally 33–35.5 cm in the newborn infant, whilst enlarging throughout infancy will gradually become more proportionate to body size. At first the cranium appears large, however this is normal in infants. Sutures between skull bones have not completely fused and this is noticeable at the anterior fontanelle, which is covered by a membrane. The posterior fontanelle usually fuses by 0–6 weeks.

Play

Starts initially as egocentric, all items being brought to the body and tested through the mouth. Gradually, as development progresses, play becomes more adventurous and the one-year-old will still seek attention to find a dropped toy, although he can now look to see where it has gone.

Sleep

There are several safety aspects associated with sleep; firstly the mattress should fit the cot sides tightly to prevent trapping the head; secondly, pillows are unsafe because of suffocation. Cots, carrycots and prams should always have the sides placed upright.

Table 8.1 Growth (average weights and sizes), mobility, play, work and sleep through the stages of development

a) Infants: 0–1 year

Growth

Height at birth	50 cm
Height at one year	75 cm
Weight at birth	3.4 kg
Weight at one year	B: 10.3 kg/G: 9.6 kg
Head circumference	33–35.5 cm

Anterior fontanelle open until 12–18 months
Posterior fontanelle fuses at 0–6 weeks

	MOBILITY	PLAY	SLEEP
1–3 months	Lies prone, hands grasped, pelvis raised. By six weeks head lifted off mattress. Following light with eyes.	Brightly coloured mobiles. Soft fluffy toys. All toys safe, bright colours and washable.	Sleeps between feeds, personal cleansing and cuddles. Approx. 18–20 hours per day.
3–6 months	Holds head upright. Rises on to wrists. Turns to sound. Laughs. Babbles. Explores everything with the mouth.	Brightly coloured noisy toys. Rattles. Activity centres. Toys that move when touched.	Awake for longer periods after feeds.
6–9 months	Rolls over from front to back. Stands up if supported. Likes mirror image. Uses a teacher beaker. Says one word.	Mirrors, bricks, musical toys.	Has periods between feeds when he lies awake content and happy. Gurgles and babbles to self. Watches and listens.
9–12 months	Sits upright without support. Holds self up when standing. Attempts to walk. Pincer grip. Says three words.	As above and Peek-a-Boo! Push-along toys.	As above.

b) Toddlers: 1–3 years

Growth

Height	85 cm
Weight at two years	B: 12.7 kg/G: 12.0 kg

By 18 months the anterior fontanelle should have fused.

MOBILITY	PLAY/WORK	SLEEP
Gross motor Walks alone. Assists	Community resources may influence work and	Needs 10–12 hours at night, e.g. 6–6.

Table 8.1 *cont.*

MOBILITY	PLAY/WORK	SLEEP
self-balance by stretching out arms and widening gait. Goes upstairs and tries to come down (can fall so gates are important). *Fine motor* Builds a tower block of bricks by two years old. Scribbles with a crayon in palm of hand.	play. Toddler clubs and nurseries may be available and encourage toddlers to gain independence, whilst learning to play together. *Key areas* Safety in play. Socialisation through play. Parallel play (playing by yourself with your own toys alongside other toddlers). Musical, noisy toys e.g. drums. Push-along toys. Trikes and cars without pedals. Building bricks. Post boxes (post plastic pieces through different holes in box). Simple games. Picture books. Water play. Has own toys.	A nap in the morning and afternoon for 1–2 hours. Gradual introduction of pillows. Watch for climbing out of cots and pushchairs, firmly 'strap in'.

c) Preschool children: 3–5 years

Growth

Height	Adds 8 cm to height each year.
Weight	Adds 2 kg and more to weight per year until five years.

MOBILITY	PLAY/WORK	SLEEP
Gross motor Climbs, hops, balances. Kicks a ball with improved balance. Goes up and down stairs in an adult fashion. Rides a trike with pedals. *Fine motor* Threads beads on to a string. Prints name, copies letters O and V.	Attendance at a day nursery may continue. There are also preschool playgroups. These community resources not only teach about play but also help the transition necessary from home to school. *Key areas* Fantasy and make-believe play. Sharing begins. Socialisation continues. Dressing up in roles, e.g. mother, father. Play at	Still requires around ten hours sleep. May need a nap in the afternoon of one or two hours. Transition from a cot to a bed may start. (In hospital cots are usually advised until five years, because of the height of the beds from the floor).

Table 8.1 *cont.*

MOBILITY	PLAY/WORK	SLEEP
	house-keeping pretend cooking & cleaning. Has own toys, talks to them and to imaginary toys and friends. Plays hide and seek. Likes group games. Likes to cut out pictures. Does 2–6 piece jigsaws. Reads simple books. Finger paints.	

d) School children: 5–11 years
Growth

Height	Gains 6.25 cm per year.
Weight	Gains 3.18 kg per year.

MOBILITY	WORK (EDUCATION)/PLAY	SLEEP
Gross motor Body is proportionate, limbs have increased muscle. Movement is steady, balanced and coordinated. Between the ages of 5 and 11 years, the child runs and jumps, skips, climbs trees. He learns to use this mobility in various sporting activities, such as school races, football and tennis. Leisure too may use this mobility, such as ballet, playing a musical instrument and riding bikes. *Fine motor* Able to print name, address and age. Manipulates objects with great dexterity. 'Dog ears', books. By the end of this period, writing is script and drawing and colouring advanced.	It is a statutory requirement to send a child to school at 5 years. It can be a difficult time for parents and child alike. However, once the child is settled, he usually enjoys a busy day. School teachers combine learning with play, the latter being familiar to the child, whilst learning reading, writing and arithmetic presents a challenge. School friends become more important often than parents and this can cause disharmony in the family. Examples of play might include acting out stories, crafts such as carpentry and needlework, outdoor play, swimming, horse-riding, card and board games.	School children tire themselves with new learning and boundless energy. 9–10 hours sleep is still advisable, in order that they may be able to cope with school. Tired children get irritable. Sleep is now in a bed.

Table 8.1 *cont.*

e) Adolescents: 11–18 years

GROWTH AND PUBERTAL CHANGES	MOBILITY	EDUCATION AND PLAY	SLEEP
Height Girls 11–14 155 cm 15–18 162.5 cm Boys 11–14 157.5 cm 15–18 172.5 cm *Weight* Girls 11–14 44 kg 15–18 54 kg Boys 11–14 44 kg 15–18 60 kg *Sexual changes* Girls–Growth spurt –Breast development –Pubic and axillary hair –Hips widen –Fat is redistributed –Commencement of the menstrual cycle Boys–Growth spurt –Testes, penis and scrotum enlarge –Chest, pubic and axillary hair –Broadening of shoulders –Elongation of limbs –Facial hair	The emphasis in mobility is in relation both to the growth spurt associated with puberty and to the mental development enhanced by school. Mobility starts off in adolescence as coordinated, but often becomes sloppy and sometimes clumsy. The latter is caused by disproportionate growth between the upper and lower parts of the body, especially in boys. The arms elongate before the legs. Round-shoulderedness in girls may be to do with hiding breast development. Mobility also relates to 'being different' which is a feature of adolescence. This is a period of strength and agility often seen in competitive sports.	School offers a challenge, and competition is encouraged through the examination system. It is important that all adolescents are seen as individuals, otherwise falling behind with work can cause stress, apathy or truancy. School should also prepare the adolescent for his future career. The GCSE exams are meant to be more realistic and in line with adult careers. With high unemployment, the motivation to do well at school may be difficult. Play at school is now formalised into regulated sports periods. Adolescents are capable of great achievement in sport. Play away from school	The adolescent's need for sleep declines by about 14 years to 8 or 8½ hours per night. Adolescents often appear tired and lazy and can 'never wake up'.

Table 8.1 *cont.*

GROWTH AND PUBERTAL CHANGES	MOBILITY	EDUCATION AND PLAY	SLEEP
–'Breaking' of the voice –Nocturnal emissions and ejaculation through masturbation		starts off with friends of the same sex, moves on to mixed groups of friends and then to single partners. Social clubs, discos and just 'hanging around' are popular.	

CHECK LIST

Assessment of the child's mobility, play and work needs and sleep

1. Ask parents what they have noted about their child's mobility, play, work and sleep patterns.
2. Note the age and stage of the child's development (infant, toddler etc.). Has any regression occurred?
3. Is mobility painful, restricted or limited because of trauma?
4. If injury is present, do the child's and the parents' stories tally?
5. What does the child play with? Has he any special toys? If so note these carefully. Does he play alone, or are there others in the family?
6. Has sleep been disturbed, as an infant or currently? Is the child more sleepy than usual?

The handicapped child

Handicapping conditions may be physical, mental or both. Some handicaps occur because of chromosomal abnormalities such as Down's syndrome, others occur due to birth trauma and anoxia, e.g. cerebral palsy. Surgery and infection may leave a child handicapped, examples of this are brain surgery for tumours and meningitis causing residual brain or other damage, e.g. deafness. Trauma may cause a handicap, such as loss of a limb. Many handicaps are of unknown origin and this makes it very difficult for parents to accept. Guilt and self-blame are often central features of parents' reactions to producing a handicapped child.

Mobilising, working, playing and sleeping in relation to the handicapped child

Many handicaps seriously limit the child's ability to mobilise and therefore affect many of the other normal activities of living. Children's development largely depends on the ability to move as well as development of the thought processes, and not least the ability to communicate.

The handicapped child as a basis for a care plan could be considered in any one of the previous chapters; however, many of the problems arising do so because the child cannot 'do' for himself and by school age this is certainly abnormal.

The school child with cerebral palsy

School children are naturally energetic, noisy, communicative and beginning to be independent. Social skills such as eliminating, cleansing, dressing, eating and drinking are established. There is a desire to learn, enhanced by school and play and increased awareness of the need for safety.

CARE PLAN

An eight-year-old boy with cerebral palsy

Consider then an eight-year-old boy with cerebral palsy, admitted to hospital following the onset of epileptic fits. This is not Paul's first admission; but one of many for the same problem. His distraught father accompanies him, continually ensuring that the nurses know exactly how to care for Paul while he is to be hospitalised. Paul's father looks tired and weary, the culmination of working and sleepless nights. He has brought Paul to hospital as his wife just cannot face going through the same traumas with Paul, yet again.

On admission Paul is sleepy, not fitting, his legs are outstretched and 'scissored' at the ankles (spasticity) and he is in wet trousers. He had one fit during the journey to hospital from his home 20 miles away.

After settling Paul in one place in the ward where he could be frequently observed and was safe, his father left to return home. The ward sister had suggested he return to his wife and to take a rest, possibly not returning for a few days, up to a week. Respite from care is essential for parents of handicapped children. Paul's father had the hospital and ward phone number and was encouraged to phone whenever he wanted.

Cerebral palsy may cover a variety of causes which have culminated in a child born with malfunction of motorcentres and pathways of the brain. Children are mentally handicapped, as well as having paralysis, weakness, incoordination and ataxia. There is little and slow progress developmentally in all aspects. Some children die early due to overwhelming infection or anoxic problems. Others live longer; however, progress and lifespan depends on the severity of cerebral palsy. The lay term for this handicap is 'spastic'.

Epilepsy is a convulsive disorder, associated with episodic disturbances of brain function. Epileptic fits, may be grand mal, petit mal, focal or myoclonic (in infants). When convulsions occur in a series, this is known as status epilepticus.

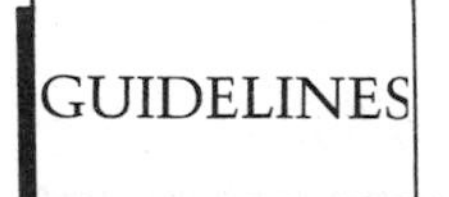

Creating a care plan

The problems identified for Paul have been prioritised using the Activities of Living framework. *The care to be given appears as headings only.* In your own paediatric area, these might be used to form the basis of a ward care plan. Not all problems will relate to all children with cerebral palsy, therefore use these as a guideline.

Table 8.2 Problems, goals and nursing care arising from difficulties with normal activities of living

PROBLEMS	GOALS AND NURSING CARE
1 **Maintaining a safe environment and breathing.** *Inability to maintain safety in relation to physical and mental development and particularly in relation to airway maintenance.*	Goals: Maintain airway and safety of the internal and external environment. Nursing care points: — Emergency equipment, oxygen and suction — Position on side — Care during epileptic fits — Administering medications — Neurological state — Safety of cot and surroundings and when out of bed — Safety with food, medicines, drink and utensils — Safety with toys — Diminished sensation e.g. pain, heat, cold — Predisposition to infection.
2 **Communicating** *Unable to speak, but understands some spoken words and gestures. Communicates non-verbally on occasions.*	Goals: Recognise methods of communication, develop these and use multidisciplinary team where applicable. Nursing care points: — Keep in touch with parents — Face child to communicate — Speak slowly and clearly — Use touch — Observe non-verbal communication and sounds from verbal communication — Speech therapy if applicable.

Table 8.2 *cont.*

PROBLEMS	GOALS AND NURSING CARE
3 **Eating and drinking** *Unable to feed self. Persistence of a bite reflex, rather than chewing. Low weight for age.*	Goals: Maintain nutrition and hydration. Set target for weight gain. Nursing care points: — Suitable diet, cut up and texture which is semi-solid — Feed child at socially acceptable times — Fluid intake — Use utensils to encourage chewing — Weigh weekly — Keep food and fluid chart.
4 **Eliminating, personal cleansing and dressing** *Unable to cleanse and dress unless performed for him. (p) for pressure sores and skin injury. Incontinent of urine. (p) for constipation.*	Goals: Maintain body cleanliness and appearance. Prevent pressure sores and constipation, also sore skin from urinary incontinence. Nursing care points: — Safe environment — Cleansing and dressing routine — Use Norton scale score assessment. Position and turn regularly (1–2 hourly) — Change nappy and wash frequently — Provide diet and medications to prevent constipation. — Bowel chart — Suppositories or enemas as prescribed.
5 **Maintaining body temperature** *(p) pyrexia due to infection (*e.g. chest or urinary*) *or* (p) lowered temperature due to lack of communication, mobility and self-care, also low BMR and poor diet.*	Goals: Maintain constant body temperature, by frequent observation and care. Provide appropriate care for lowered or raised temperature. Nursing care points: — See Eliminating, personal cleansing and dressing. Also: Maintaining a safe environment and breathing; Eating and drinking; Mobilising — Monitoring body temperature daily if no problems.

Table 8.2 *cont.*

PROBLEMS	GOALS AND NURSING CARE
6 **Mobilising, working, playing and sleeping** *Unable to move around, educationally subnormal, unable to play alone. Disturbed sleep pattern.*	Goals: Provide appropriate stimulation through play and contact Routine established for mobility and rest. Nursing care points: — Safety — Put limbs through a range of movements several times a day — Involve physiotherapist — Prevent 'scissoring' of legs — Place in a position where other children can be seen — Suitable play items — Spend time playing — Schooling (see below) — Rest periods in the day may be needed.
7 **Expressing sexuality** *Altered body image, but normal external physical development*	Goals: Promote normal sexuality i.e. dress as a boy, give toys which a boy would like, etc. Nursing care points: — Privacy at all times — Clothes — Toys — Try to encourage a normal routine for child.
8 **Dying** *Parents' fear of the child dying*	Goals: Minimise anxiety during this admission by communication. Nursing care points: — Refer to Chapter 10, The dying child.

EVALUATION

Each of the goals set and the care given need evaluating at least daily. The alteration to problems of a handicapped child are slow and daily evaluation may not show progress. However, it is important to note if nursing care has been effective and of course, to be able to report to the parents any changes the child has made. For parents every tiny step is an important one and this should be remembered when planning nursing care, so that the handicapped child does not regress while in hospital.

Community and educational facilities

Community facilities

Relatives, friends and neighbours; health visitor or district (community) nurse; clinical nurse specialists; physiotherapists; speech therapists; occupational therapists; general practitioners; genetic counsellors; antenatal clinics and midwives; nursery schools; local government through the social worker for aids to living, e.g. utensils, wheelchairs etc., and housing alterations, financial assistance; DHSS benefits; self-help and support groups; transport assistance; holidays for children or respite homes; residential care; employment through the disablement resettlement officer; fund-raising activities.

Education

Special schools may be used for educating handicapped children, or special classes in ordinary schools. Sometimes handicapped children are better in an ordinary day school. Adaptation of ordinary schools may include ramps for wheelchairs, wide classroom doors and suitable seating. The school teacher should be aware of what is wrong with the child and how to act in an emergency (e.g. an epileptic fit). There are some specially trained teachers who, for instance, visit the blind or deaf child at home. The school nurse and doctor should closely monitor the mental and physical development of the handicapped child at school.

REFERENCES

FRANKENBURG, W. K. & DODDS, J. B. 1969. *The Denver Developmental Screening Test (DDST).* University of Colorado Medical Centre.

NORTON, D., MCLAREN, R. & EXTON-SMITH, A. N. 1975. *An Investigation of Geriatric Nursing Problems in Hospital.* Churchill Livingstone, Edinburgh.

FURTHER READING

BATEMAN, H. 1987. Fun and Games. *Community Outlook*, (April), 12–23.

BEE, H. 1985. *The Developing Child*, 4th Edn. Harper & Row, New York.

BOWLEY, A. H. & GARDNER, L. 1980. *The Handicapped Child: Educational and psychological guidance for the organically handicapped*, 4th Edn. Churchill Livingstone, Edinburgh.

Life Cycle Series published 1979–1980:

CONGER, J. *Adolesence: Generation under pressure.*

RICHARDS, M. *Infancy: World of the newborn.*

WHITE, S. & WHITE, B. N. *Childhood: Pathways of discovery.* Harper & Row, London.

PARRISH, A. & COLLINS, S. (Eds). 1987. *Mental Handicap.* The Essentials of Nursing Series. Macmillan Education, London.

RENWICK, J. 1987. Child's Play. *Community Outlook*, (April), 20–21.

RUSSELL, P. 1984. *The Wheelchair Child*, 2nd Edn. The Human Horizon Series. Souvenir Press, London.

SHERIDAN, M. D. 1977. *Spontaneous Play in Early Childhood: 0–5 years.* NFER Publications, Windsor.

SHERIDAN, M. D. 1984. *From birth to 5 years*, Children's Developmental Progress. NFER Publications, Windsor.

SPECIAL EDUCATIONAL NEEDS. 1978. *Committee of inquiry into the education of handicapped children and young people.* Chairman: Warnock, H. M. HMSO, London.

9 Expressing sexuality

In this chapter consideration is given to the child's developing sexuality, both emotionally and physically, as well as alterations in the child's body image. How the child learns about his body both internally and externally will help him in identifying both his body boundaries and body functions and contribute to his understanding of sexuality. Many aspects of this topic are reflected in other activities of living, such as changes in body structure and function as noted in Chapters 4 and 8, differences in cleansing, dressing and eliminating in Chapter 7 and toys and playthings in Chapter 8.

To illustrate care of a child with an altered body image, an exercise is included for you to complete about a preschooler of four years old with burns to his abdomen and lower chest.

Further consideration is given to the difficult and emotive topic of child sexual abuse.

Health promotion and education

Infants

Infants are treated as male or female from birth, in that they are given a name according to their gender. In language, infants are taught whether they are 'he' or 'she' and sayings such as 'that's a good boy or girl' reinforce the gender role.

When the infant is handled, girls are likely to be treated more tenderly, whilst infant boys are often handled boisterously and encouraged to be very active in response. Until recent years, traditionally pink clothes and bedding were for girls and blue for boys. With the advent of chain stores specifically for infants and young children, colours in which to dress children are wide-ranging and less sexually orientated. Young infants are invariably dressed alike whether male or female, both being dressed, for example, in babygros.

Most infants are given cuddly, bright and mobile toys at first and there appears to be no delineation between the sexes.

The infant considers himself part of his main caregiver, usually his mother, and therefore he is unaware of his body boundaries and also that he has a particular body image. All new things are tested through the mouth and gradually he learns to use and explore with his hands and then his legs. Older infants touch their genitals, not as a deliberate sexual act, but because when they discover that part of their body, touching provides a pleasurable experience.

Toddlers

By the time the child is two years old, he can identify others as boys or girls by their external appearance.

In Western culture evidence of promotion of sexual identity becomes stronger. Social stereotyping is often inadvertently introduced into the young child's life through language, toys, clothing and so on.

The child is also realising that he is a separate being from his parents, both physically and psychologically. This in turn will develop his body image, but as yet he cannot localise body parts, pain being an example of this.

Preschool children

By the time the child is three years old, he knows whether he is a boy or girl and he wants to know how the other sex works, for instance, how girls can urinate without a penis.

Preschool children want to know where *they* came from and questions such as 'where do babies come from' are not unusual at this age. Honest explanations have to be given rather than making a fuss, or avoiding answering. Ultimately children will explore their genitals to find out for themselves how babies are born: how does a baby as big as they are pass through such a small opening? It is also not unusual for preschoolers to masturbate. Freud called the stages between three and six years the genital/phallic stage. This in part relates to the development of sexual awareness, but also links to the vivid imagination of preschoolers. Freud also suggests that the child forms an attachment to the parent of the opposite sex – the Oedipal phase.

Play now becomes more masculine or feminine. Girls are encouraged to and engage in domesticated play such as cooking, and often they also like dressing up and playing with dolls. Boys on the other hand, are encouraged to play with trucks and bricks, their play being more physically active and aggressive, and it seems more acceptable for them to fight and shout during play.

The preschooler is very certain of his body boundaries and does not like any invasive procedures. Injections, venepuncture and cuts (wounds) to the body are examples. Because he is aware of his skin being the external part of him, he thinks any puncture of this will allow his insides to 'leak out'. Combined with this is a fear of intrusion to his genital region, therefore examinations and investigations should be kept to a minimum. If they are necessary they need careful explanation, often using dolls or toys first. The literal thought processes of the preschooler also contribute to his concern about intrusion to his body. If he has to have things 'taken away' or 'fixed', this is a cause of great stress. Jolly (1977) suggests that children can be given diagrams to explain parts of the body before operation. The children can be asked what part of the body is to be mended? They can also help parents understand. Jolly also discusses how children in a burns unit in the USA were helped to work through their terrible alteration to body image. Using a doll, a trained nurse asked the child how the doll felt. She then gave the child scissors to cut out the 'skin' of the doll, where it hurt. In almost every case, the child removed the 'skin' from the doll in the same area as where they had been burned. The doll was then kept for the treatment and care which would be necessary for the child.

School children

Parents and school teachers too often make clear their sexual role expectations of the child. Girls are told not to be 'tomboys' and boys not to be 'sissy'.

Children will eventually style themselves after the parent of the same sex; in other words they achieve a sexual identity role. There is a continuation at the beginning of school age, around five years, of exploring sexual body parts. Children indulge in 'doctor play' with each other, to discover each others' sexual identity. Girls may investigate their body to find out where babies come from and are often scolded if caught doing so. By the middle school years, sex education can begin formally. Most girls are beginning to understand the growth of babies inside mothers. Smutty jokes are told by the age of eight years and by nine, girls know about menstruation and boys show interest in their father's reproductive organs and sexuality. Some girls will have entered the pubertal period by the age of nine or ten.

Towards the end of the school years, and before adolescence, there is either interest or disinterest in the opposite sex. Children know about sexual intercourse and often regard this as nasty. Girls may have breast development and boys erections. With these physical changes, girls either become interested in their body or very embarrassed. Boys seem interested in the bodily changes of girls, which can of course make them more embarrassed.

Muller *et al.* (1986) suggest that early friendships show little evidence of sex preferences, but that by 11 years sex segregation is almost total.

School teachers contribute to sex segregation from an early age by using class registers and dividing up the sexes in sports and class activities.

General trends from the National Child Development Study Findings (Fogelman 1983) noted that educationally, school children differed little in achievement according to gender, at the age of seven years and again at 11 years. However, by 16 years boys had moved ahead in mathematics.

Quiggin (1977) followed up early research about children's knowledge of their internal body parts by studying a group of 11-year-olds. Previous studies of four- to eight-year-olds had shown that children think of their bodies as hollow organs with reservoirs for food, waste and blood. Nine- to eleven-year-olds thought that body parts which could be felt were larger than those which had little or no sensation. The most commonly named organs were the heart, brain and bones.

In Quiggin's study, it was found that boys named and drew more muscle and bone structure, e.g. the leg muscles, pelvis and jaw. Girls named and drew tonsils, adenoids, uterus, cells, calves, veins and ribs. Arbitrary conclusions from his study suggest that boys are concerned with body framework and muscle development, in keeping with male sexual identity.

A study in 1973 by Fleming noted that children drew their 'ill' organ or a disabled body part bigger than other parts. In some cases of handicap, the deformed or ill part was all that was drawn. It is also interesting to note how school children link up illness with alteration to their body.

Wood (1983) suggests that children who fall into the age group below six years old think that illness is due to infection. The seven-to eleven-year-old groups ('concrete operations' in Piaget's phases) cited several reasons for illness. The most commonly chosen cause was self-action or blame. Others included outside forces, traumatic injury, infection and uncrystallised ideas. In children over ten years, the 'germ theory' was often stated as the cause of illness. In children over 12 years, multiple factors were believed to lead to illness. Wood noted that previous experience such as trauma affected the child's choice of reason; in this case an outside force was seen to cause illness.

Jolly (1985) suggests that children don't talk or write about the actual illness or accident which took them to hospital. Stories stop short of the actual details of the illness, as if it is too stressful for the child to recall. Children do recall invasive procedures such as injections and when they have been caused to have pain.

Adolescents

By the time the child reaches adolescence, he has either been through or is about to undergo the immense changes to his body associated with puberty. These changes occur due to a surge of reproductive hormones, which may start as early as nine years in girls and several years later in boys. Details of body changes are discussed on page 140 and are included in Chapter 8.

During this time of developing sexual maturity and independence, experimentation and family conflict can occur. There is a strong attraction for the opposite sex, enhanced by bodily changes. Adolescents can feel strange about these changes, either accentuating or hiding them. For instance, girls may wear tight clothes to show off their figure, alternatively they may become round-shouldered or wear baggy clothes to hide their body contours. For boys, there is often little control over erections and subsequent emissions, particularly at night. Whilst the feelings associated with this are pleasant, socially they must be controlled.

Adolescents who do not reach puberty at the same time as their peers are often teased and made to feel isolated. This appears to affect boys particularly. Girls, on the other hand, often compare their rate of development with each other.

Thus, the combination of body changes, self and sexual awareness and sexual urge consolidates the adolescent's sex role identity. It is often a stormy time, both for parents and the adolescent. Boys seem more concerned with the physical gratification associated with sex, girls more often relate their feelings to love. Adolescents indulge in petting and sexual experimentation. At first pairs are formed within a group, later pairs will go out together without the group. By the end of adolescence, hetero- or homosexual relationships have been formed by a large percentage of people.

Parents have tried to support and educate through this period and to prepare the adolescent for marriage and family life. There is also role preparation for employment. More recently, this has been less sexually orientated, although there are still many occupations which appear exclusive to one or other sex. (Think about nursing, which is still a female-dominated occupation.)

SEX EDUCATION

Educating children about sexual changes is a very personal subject. Some parents start this early, others wait until puberty and some parents let the school educate the child, or indeed, let the child find out for himself. Professionals who may be involved in explaining sexual changes are the health visitor, who may visit schools, and the school nurse and school teacher who may give lessons; however, often parental consent is needed before the child may attend sex education classes. Ultimately, how much the child may learn in a formal setting is controlled by parents.

Mothers have expectations that their daughters will talk to and learn from them. Boys pick up information in a more casual manner. Overall most learning about sexual identity is gained from parents, books, television and friends in and out of the school.

Developmental aspects

Foetal development

During foetal life the infant's sex has been determined, along with other genetic characteristics. Boys have an XY sex chromosome and girls an XX chromosome. Along with the sex chromosomes, external and internal physical features develop, which determine the sex of the child.

By the time the male infant is born, testes should be in the scrotum and the epididymis, vas deferens and seminal vesicles formed internally. Externally boys should have a penis.

Girls are born with a uterus, ovaries, fallopian tubes and vagina internally and labial folds, clitoris and vaginal opening externally. Sometimes female infants appear to have swollen labia until the hormonal balance in the body adjusts to extra-uterine life.

Infants

Unless any defects have occurred, all physical characteristics relating to sexual development should be properly formed and present at birth. Occasionally, the testes are slow to descend in the male infant. If this persists then surgery may be necessary. Sexual anatomy will grow during the early years until puberty, when considerable changes take place. The sexuality of the infant becomes apparent through his facial appeal and through the way he is dressed and handled.

Toddlers, preschool and school children

There is little change to sexual characteristics physically during the toddler to school child age. Obviously the gender of the child becomes more accentuated through clothes and play and so on. During late school age and early adolescence many children are prepubertal or pubertal.

Adolescents

During the pubertal stage which precedes and heralds the onset of adolescence, there is a surge of sex hormones. These give rise to the sexual changes indicated in Table 9.1.

These major physical changes for male and female are in part responsible for the psychological changes noted in the adolescent. Body image is totally altered and it takes time for the adolescent to adjust. Friends and peers can be both a source of comfort and also be unkind. Boys may become awkward and clumsy because of disproportionate growth of arms and legs. Girls may put on 'puppy fat' until hormonal balance has been restored.

Table 9.1 Physical changes associated with puberty in boys and girls

BOYS (12–14 years)	GIRLS (10–12 years)
Hormone change: rise in testosterone production	Hormone change: rise in oestrogen production
Height growth spurt	Height growth spurt
Testes, scrotum and penis enlarge	Breast development
Pubic, chest and axillary hair	Pubic and axillary hair
Limbs elongate, shoulders broaden	Broadening of the hips
Facial hair appears	Fat redistribution
Deepening of voice – 'voice breaks'	Commencement of the menstrual cycle
Ejaculation often at night or by masturbation	Underarm perspiration
Underarm perspiration	Acne on the face
Acne on the face	

CHECK LIST

Assessment of the child's sexuality

1 Has the child any special names for his sexual organs?
2 Note how the parents address, clothe and play with the child.
3 Ensure that privacy is available (and let the child and parents know this) for elimination, cleansing and dressing.
4 Does the child have something to say about his body image (e.g. he doesn't want holes put in his skin)?
5 At what stage of puberty is the late school child or adolescent? This may be difficult information to obtain but use observational skills and build up a relationship with the child or adolescent to find out.
6 Are there any problems associated with sexuality, e.g. physical defects, dislike of one parent, signs of sexual abuse?

EXERCISE

A four-year-old preschooler with burns to his abdomen and lower chest

The selection of a preschool child with burns to illustrate an altered sexuality state, reflects

Fig. 9.1 Diagram to assess percentage of body burned

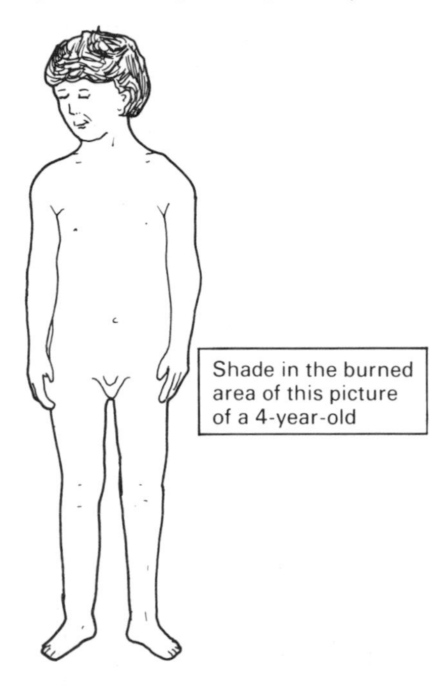

knowledge also gained in other chapters. When considering the burned child, safety and the environment (Chapter 2), pain and communication (Chapter 3), fluid balance (Chapter 6), elimination, personal cleansing and dressing (Chapter 7), mobility and play (Chapter 8), and observations (Chapters 4 and 5) all contribute to the nursing care.

1 Identify at least *four factors* which could have caused burns to the abdomen and lower chest of a four-year-old child.
2 Using the diagram in Fig. 9.1, shade in the affected area and state the percentage of the body involved (burned) in a four-year-old child.
3 The diagram represents one way of medically assessing a child's burns.

Identify *two other* types of assessment of burns which the medical staff will use.

4 In adults the 'rule of nine' is used to assess the burned area. State *one* reason why this assessment is not totally suitable for young children.

5 *Where* would you expect to nurse this four-year-old burned child? State why this type of nursing is necessary.

6 The main problems which the four-year-old child will present with on arrival to the paediatric ward are as follows:

   (i) *Fluid loss*, due to seepage of fluid from the burned area. This will also alter the fluid balance of the body and affect pulse, BP and respirations; these may also be associated with hypovolaemic shock.

   (ii) *Pain*, due to damaged nerve endings.

   (iii) *Anxiety*, due to accident, emergency treatment, pain and hospitalisation.

   At four years old, the child will not understand what has happened and will be very distraught.

   Question (i): Fluid loss

   a) What type of observations should be made, how often and why?

   b) Why must a very careful check be kept on the intravenous fluids being infused?

   Question (ii): Pain

   a) How could you assess pain in a four-year-old?

   b) Why is it important to give analgesia?

   c) Which route of administration for analgesia is the doctor likely to prescribe? Try to give some rationale for this.

Question (iii): Anxiety

a) What can be done immediately and in the long term to lessen anxiety in the four-year-old?

b) To what is it likely that a four-year-old attributes his burns?

7 Name at least three other potential (p) problems which may occur in the immediate period following burns.

8 Suggest one way in which play can be used to help the burned child overcome fear and anxiety.

9 In the long term, the four-year-old is likely to have a degree of scarring on his abdomen and chest. What psychological scars is the child likely to have in the future?

10 If you noticed burns on a child which did not relate to an accident, hospital admission, etc., how would you handle the situation?

Child sexual abuse

In Chapter 2, a brief outline of child abuse and paediatric care was given. In this section, the increasing problem of sexual abuse of children is explored more fully.

Sexual abuse of children, particularly incest, is not new in society. Various cultures in ancient times actually encouraged incest to maintain 'purity of lineage' in royal families. However, current values in society have brought this problem under scrutiny, as well as television documentaries and other media attention. 'Childwatch' helpline exposed a subject which for years had been well hidden.

Kempe and Kempe (1978) defined the sexual exploitation of children as 'the involvement of dependent, developmentally immature children and adolescents in sexual activities that they do not fully comprehend, to which they are unable to give informed consent, and that violate the social taboos of family roles'.

There is no doubt that most people feel disgust and anger when children are sexually abused. Thus paediatric nurses faced with these children in outpatients, accident and emergency and childrens' wards, may expect to have similar emotions to come to terms with themselves before being able to feel comfortable with looking after such a family.

A considerable number of sexually abused children are never seen in any clinic or department. The NSPCC (1985) reports that sexual abuse accounts for 17.8% of the total number of children abused. The reporting of all abuse cases has increased most in the sexual abuse category.

Vousden (1987) discusses some of the reasons why sexual exploitation occurs. Marital problems, divorce and societal changes have probably led to the increase in this sort of abuse. If changes in the family structure are set in the context of high unemployment, debts and poor housing, it becomes possible to see how any sort of child abuse can occur. However, sexual abuse goes much deeper into family relationships and particularly those where it is the father abusing the daughter and where the wife may be disillusioned with the marriage and actually knows that her daughter is being exploited by her husband.

The NSPCC has a key role in training professionals to observe for sexual abuse, also it disseminates educative information and keeps a non-accidental injury register. Amongst those whom the society trains are playgroup workers. Other professionals who must be well informed are medical staff, health visitors, ward nursing staff, school nurses, school teachers and social workers. The police are also often involved and have recently developed a more sensitive approach to this dilemma, by having specially trained constables (often women) to carry out necessary interviews with children. The use of dolls has been introduced for children to use to assist the explanation of what has been done to them. In criminal courts, children are protected from seeing the abuser and the use of one-way mirrors and video recordings has recently been employed. There is a move towards believing the child's evidence, although currently there is no law that it will necessarily be accepted or used. It should be noted that incest is a criminal offence and if a doctor suspects a child has been sexually abused, he should notify the police and involve the social services.

If sexual abuse is suspected, this provisional diagnosis is based on several features. Firstly, that the child's story should be believed. Secondly that physical injury to the genitalia and anal areas is not usually caused by 'natural' accidents, e.g. falling on a railing. A careful and sensitive interview and examination is given to the child, establishing if there are any other external features such as bruises or bites. The child's underclothes are checked for blood and semen. The parents will also need careful handling and should be interviewed separately, so that any family ties can be maintained rather than further destroyed.

It is usual that a case conference is held within 72 hours of a child being admitted to hospital (or a foster home). Representatives include medical and nursing staff, social services, health visitors and the NSPCC and police where applicable. So that the family has time to sort out the impact which the discovery of incest may have on already strained relationships, *and* so that the child is protected, a Place of Safety order is usually sought from a magistrate. This order lasts for 28 days and during this time the child may not be removed from the designated safe place. This is the point at which most paediatric nurses come into contact with sexually abused children, unless they have been working in children's clinics or paediatric casualty.

The role of the paediatric nurse, as in any form of abuse, is to observe the child and family, especially their relationships. The child may find it difficult to relate to nursing staff and despite being abused, may still turn to his visiting parents for comfort. Any physical or psychological changes which are noted must be reported to the nurse in charge.

Several case conferences are usually necessary before a decision on the child's future can be made. If a crime is suspected, then criminal proceedings may necessitate the child remaining in a safe environment for some time. Ultimately the child may need fostering or may be returned home, with supervision from the social services and health visitor.

This topic causes nursing staff considerable emotional distress, and as a student nurse, you will need time and support to sort out your personal feelings when nursing sexually abused children.

REFERENCES

FLEMING, J. W. 1973. Understanding hospitalised children through drawings (8th Nursing Research Conference in New Mexico). Abstracted in *Nursing Research*, **22**, 1:(88) Abs. 86.

FOGELMAN, K. (Ed). 1983. *Growing up in Great Britain*. Papers from the National Child Development Study. Macmillan for NCB, London.

FREUD, S. 1983. In *Introduction to Psychology*, 8th Edn. Hilgard, Atkinson & Atkinson (Eds). Harcourt Brace Jovanovich, New York.

JOLLY, J. 1985. Child Health: Timmy goes to hospital. *Nursing Times*, **81**(13), 27–30.

JOLLY, J. D. 1977. How to be in hospital without being frightened. *Nursing Times*, **73**(1853), 1887–1888.

KEMPE, R. S. & KEMPE, C. 1978. *Child Abuse*. Open University Press, Milton Keynes.

MCAREE, J. 1987. Child Abuse: A family affair. *Nursing Times*, **83**(6), 26–30.

MULLER, D. J., HARRIS, P. J. & WATTLEY, L. 1986. *Nursing Children: Psychology, Research and Practice*. Lippincott Nursing Series. Harper & Row, London.

QUIGGIN, V. 1977. Children's knowledge of their internal body parts. *Nursing Times*, **73**(1135), 1146–1151.

VOUSDEN, M. 1987. Child abuse behind closed doors. *Nursing Times*, **83**(16), 25–26.

WOOD, S. 1983. School aged children's perceptions of the causes of illness. *Paediatric Nursing*, **9**(2), 101–104.

FURTHER READING

JONES, D. M. (Ed). 1982. *Understanding Child Abuse*. Teach Yourself Books. Hodder & Stoughton, London.

PITHERS, D. & GREENE, S. 1986. *We can say NO*. A Child's Guide (in association with NCH). Beaver Books, London.

SWANWICK, M. & OLIVER, R. 1985. Psychological Adjustment in Adolescence. *Nursing, 2nd Series*, **40** (August), 1179–1181.

10 The dying child

Coping with death and dying in any area of nursing is a difficult and emotional subject for many nurses. Because of the innocence and immaturity of children, death may be particularly hard to understand and be a very painful topic for nurses to explore.

Examining one's own feelings, whilst being very stressful, can be helpful should the death of a child occur during the paediatric experience.

Families have wide and varying beliefs about child care, but usually know what they want when their child dies. Cultural and spiritual values must be recognised, as well as each family's individual response to bereavement.

In order to support the child and his family at this distressing time, you will need guidance and supervision from experienced nursing and medical staff. However, the ability to listen and to offer a comforting hand, as well as taking the time to spend with such families, is within the realms of the student nurse. Do not get anxious if you feel you are unable to do this – you too are an individual.

The child dying from a terminal illness

An eleven-year-old with a malignant tumour

Joanne had been an alert and lively school child until the age of nine, when she complained of a swollen and painful abdomen, tiredness, nausea and generally feeling unwell. This was most out of character, as Joanne could be relied upon to join in all activities and was a motivated pupil at school. Her parents had high hopes for her future. Joanne lived at home with her mother, father, sister Suzy aged eight years and brother Rory aged five and a half years. The family appeared to get on well together and had the usual family ups and downs.

Joanne was admitted to hospital when she was nine years old and after many investigations, she was diagnosed as having a malignant growth in her abdomen. Extensive surgery followed by chemotherapy was carried out, in the hope of removing the tumour and preventing secondary deposits of malignant cells. Joanne's parents were devastated by the diagnosis, and as the surgery and treatment had to be performed quickly, they had little time to make any personal or psychological adjustments. The grieving process is not reserved only for when a person dies, but is also applicable when a disease process is diagnosed, especially when cancer is the cause. Joanne's parents were shocked and very upset and turned to each other and the nursing staff for comfort. Searching questions such as whether Joanne should be told her diagnosis, what to tell Suzy and Rory, what caused the growth and what is the prognosis? were typical and needed addressing. (See p. 173 for further consideration of the grieving process.)

After a lengthy stay in hospital, Joanne was discharged home, with contact to be made with the GP and community nurse, as well as very regular outpatient appointments and investigations at the hospital. Her parents knew that it was possible the cancer had spread elsewhere and that Joanne only had a limited lifespan.

During the next year Joanne made progress,

recovering well due to her natural resilience and the positive attitude of her parents. She returned to school, where she was welcomed back, however sports and physical activities had to be very minimal.

Her tenth birthday came and went with a big party, followed by a year of ups and downs, when Joanne sometimes felt well and at other times needed to stay at home. Her eleventh birthday was quieter, Joanne felt nauseous, very tired and expressed a wish to her mother that her birthday was just for the family. Her parents were very worried at the change in Joanne and sought medical advice. They asked for Joanne to be admitted to hospital and Joanne was in agreement with this.

After considerable investigations and discussion with parents, the medical staff felt they were unable to give any further successful treatment and that Joanne was now terminally ill.

The last episode

Joanne's parents, whilst shielding themselves from the prospect of their daughter dying, suspected that this outcome would come quickly.

Once in hospital Joanne deteriorated rapidly, losing weight, becoming very sleepy and, despite medications, frequently vomiting. It was felt necessary to insert an intravenous infusion to provide her with some fluid and to pass a naso-gastric tube, which could be aspirated when she felt sick and also to prevent inhalation of vomit. Pain control was achieved with controlled drugs and Joanne was regularly assessed to ensure pain relief was adequate. Joanne's parents became resident, taking turns to be there and at home. They were encouraged to offer as much care as they felt able, with support from the staff. Care of Joanne's pressure areas, personal cleansing and dressing and taking her to the toilet were some of these aspects.

Suzy and Rory were obviously concerned and Rory, a bit jealous about the attention Joanne was receiving. Both children needed to be told the truth, but in a way each could understand (see p. 171 children's perception of death). Siblings should be involved and allowed to visit; this will help both the dying child and the siblings themselves.

Joanne however, at 11 years old was well able to comprehend death (see p. 172). With considerable help from paediatric nursing and medical staff, when Joanne voiced some thoughts about her illness her parents were able to discuss her impending death. Later, a TV programme which touched on this subject caused all the family who had been watching it to cry and hug each other.

A child is likely to go through the stages of dying as outlined by Kubler-Ross (1976) – denial, anger, bargaining, depression and acceptance. For Joanne, these stages had probably commenced when she realised how ill she was after the first hospital admission. Her parents suspected she knew she would die, but was not prepared to discuss the subject until faced with impending death. One evening, Joanne lapsed into semi-consciousness, having spent a lovely afternoon with all the family, including a visit from Grandad. Her parents cuddled and talked softly to her. A paediatric nurse spent the evening in the room with parents and as requested the hospital chaplain had made several visits. Joanne slipped peacefully into death at 8 p.m.

Her parents and Suzy and Rory cried a lot and said their goodbyes. Mum and Dad and the nurse washed and dressed Joanne in her favourite clothes and ensured that her favourite record was in her hands.

The medical and nursing staff spent time

with the parents until they felt ready to return to a nearby guesthouse, where they had booked in. The parents would return for several days whilst details of the funeral were made. Later they would collect Joanne's personal possessions.

The staff on the ward were naturally upset and whilst dealing with this in their own ways, they also appreciated sessions which were arranged to discuss their feelings. Several nurses attended Joanne's funeral.

The story illustrates how one child died; no two children will be the same. However there are relevant points, such as stages and perceptions of death, and coping with parents and siblings, which pertain to many families. Some of these are explored later.

Death following an acute illness

When acute illness causes death, the child, the family and the team (nursing and medical) have no time for preparation. In many ways, this situation is harder to deal with, despite the fact that a lengthy emotional and stressful period has not taken place.

Parents are shocked and then guilt-ridden. 'If only . . .', 'what if . . .' are typical reactions. The grieving process can only start after the event and families need support for some time, often years. Besides funeral arrangements, there often has to be a post mortem, which can cause further distress to the family. Overall, there is suddenly an unexpected void in the family and despite being devastated, parents have to explain to siblings, relatives and friends and this is no easy task when you are trying to cope with your own grief. Parents sometimes blame each other and drift apart. It takes great strength to work through this stressful period after a child's death.

Children dying in the intensive care unit (ITU)

Causes of death
(i) Terminal illness Some examples include: leukaemic relapse; malignancy, e.g. abdominal tumour; heart disease or defects; cystic fibrosis; degenerative disorders, e.g. neurological.
(ii) Acute illness Some congenital deformities; trauma, e.g. accidents and burns; electrolyte and fluid imbalance in young children; infections, e.g. meningitis.

Children who are admitted or transferred to the ITU, may themselves not be totally aware of their surroundings. For parents, not only have they to cope with the sick child, but also with a highly technical and stressful environment. Life-saving measures override all other aspects of care and parents can feel isolated and useless. Their child has probably become unconscious, so that they do not even have the pleasure of talking to their offspring.

Other emergencies arise in ITU and parents witness what happens. Sometimes parents can draw strength from talking to each other. More often, they are lonely.

Death in this highly charged environment can be very sterile and technical, but parents need as much, if not more support to cope with the child's death. Ideally paediatric nursing and medical staff should be involved in the care of this child in the ITU.

The child's perception of death

Infants, toddlers and preschool children up to the age of three

Death is not comprehended, as this age group do not understand the life–death continuum. At toddler and preschool ages, children dislike upset to routine and ritual and will continue to do things such as save a seat at the lunch table for a family member who has died.

Preschool children 3–5 years

There is a literal interpretation of death, heard in such sayings as 'Grandpa is dead, he went to heaven'.

There is no real understanding of the meaning of death, as it cannot happen to him (the child). Often the child links death with magical thought and fantasy.

If a child of this age is dying, remember that illness, pain and separation may be viewed as punishment for being naughty. So death may be viewed this way too.

School children 5–10/11 years

The school child is concerned with how death happens, and the difference between being alive and dead.

Fears of death begin to emerge, such as horror of pain, mutilation and frightening mysteries. Death may occur violently, a concept to which TV programmes often subscribe with 'cops and robbers' series.

School children need to be helped to differentiate between death and going to sleep, otherwise they may never want to sleep. Many children of this age have lost an elderly family member or a pet and draw on these personal experiences to understand death.

Questions may be asked about what funerals are, how post mortems are carried out and so on. Children should not be excluded from funerals, but the situation should be carefully considered before the actual day.

Because of emerging fears, school children can be difficult to nurse when dying, as they ask searching questions, such as 'Am I going to die?'.

Adolescents 11–18 years

Adolescence is probably the most difficult stage for dying. Nursing this age group needs time and experience. An adolescent comprehends the process of death, but does not consider it happening to him, his family or friends. Life is for living, idealising and working out one's place in the world. Death is not for him.

Death is feared because the adolescent has not realised his full potential, because it may also distort his body image, cause dependence on others and loss of his social environment. Friends may withdraw because they cannot cope with the impending death.

An adolescent may show great resentment and have moods of anger and bitterness, through which he needs support and should not be isolated.

Stages of grief and dying

The stages outlined below (Kubler-Ross 1976) pertain both to the child who is dying and to the grieving family.

Stages and reactions

1 Denial. Shock. Disbelief.
2 Anger. Rage. Hostility.
3 Bargaining.
4 Depression.
5 Acceptance.

The speed at which each person may reach and pass through each stage is very individual.

Remember that siblings' concepts of death must be viewed also within the grieving process. They should not be 'left out', or have the truth hidden from them.

Hints which may assist when nursing a dying child

1 Teamwork and communication are essential. This includes nursing and medical staff, parents, paramedical and ancillary staff.
2 Primary nursing may be advocated, with students working in an associate or supervised role.

3 Nursing dying children can be an emotional and stressful experience. Don't be frightened of your own reactions, and seek help if you need it.
4 Tell children the truth, providing the parents have stated they want this. Children often know what they can cope with, which is often more than adults think they can. Use reflective techniques when asked a difficult question. Use parents to communicate to child.
5 Spend time with parents, just being there.
6 Involve siblings both with their brother or sister and in the normal activities in the ward.
7 Use play, art or TV programmes or books for the child to show how he feels if he cannot communicate this verbally.
8 Keep the child in touch with the outside world, with friends, school and fashions.

Spiritual and cultural needs

When someone is dying the family often turn to a spiritual leader for comfort. This is natural, as here is someone who can pave the way to death and the possible 'hereafter'. Some parents do not want contact with religion and their wishes should be noted.

Children can be christened in hospital and receive communion (if confirmed) or the last rites. Most hospitals have ministers of different denominations who can be contacted as necessary.

Cultural differences, whilst affecting many activities of living, are often accentuated at the child's death. Some cultures like peace and quiet, others need to weep and wail over the dead child. In other instances, only special people may wash the body. Consult your Health Authority Policy for specific details.

Dying at home or in a hospice

Where parents feel well supported, the dying child can be nursed at home. It is nice for him to be surrounded by a familiar environment. Sometimes parents take children home from hospital just before they die. Martinson (1980) described a study where children who were dying were nursed at home and highlighted the fact that families cannot be left alone to cope. Medical and nursing staff must be very regular visitors and be prepared to spend considerable time with the family. These personnel must also be on call to the family. Clinical nurse specialists, terminal care support teams, health visitors, paediatric community nurses and general practitioners are just some of the personnel who may take on this role. Contact with hospital and the paediatrician must be maintained.

Helen House in Oxford was the first hospice to be opened in England for terminally ill children. It caters mainly for children with neurological and metabolic diseases, however any child can be cared for who is terminally ill, even when it is known they will return home to die.

Helping the bereaved family

Contact with the paediatric ward may continue for years after the child's death. When personal possessions are collected from the ward this should be done sensitively. Items should not be bundled up and shoved in a bag for the parents. Whilst community personnel are actively involved in helping bereaved parents, several organisations exist specifically for this purpose, including: The Compassionate Friends; Parents' Lifeline; societies such as The Foundation for the Study of Infant

Deaths, The Leukaemic Society and The Lisa Sainsbury Foundation (see pp. 181–182).

The most difficult times are likely to be anniversaries, of birthdays, special days and the death of the child. The child will never be forgotten, but grief may ease over a period of time.

Sudden infant death syndrome

This syndrome has received considerable attention over the last few years. Sudden infant death syndrome (SIDS, or 'cot death') is when there is the sudden death of an apparently normal infant.

Whaley and Wong (1983) state that the death usually occurs when the child is asleep in his cot at home. Death is silent, which may be compatible with a blocked airway.

The peak age is 10–12 weeks of age with most deaths occurring before the age of six months. Premature babies may be more prone to SIDS and low socio-economic status and respiratory tract infection may be predisposing factors. Breast feeding does not necessarily prevent sudden infant death.

Possible causes are suffocation, electrolyte imbalance and apnoea. At post mortem, often no cause is found. Where a child has had apnoea attacks, parents may use an apnoea monitor at home.

Parents feel totally responsible and guilty when this traumatic death occurs. As with terminal illness, parents need to say 'goodbye' to their infant, to grieve and to be treated sensitively. Because a life was short, it does not mean that grief is also minimal. Funeral arrangements need to be made and a coroner's inquest will be necessary. The Foundation for the Study of Infant Deaths is both supportive and tries to research the cause of these sudden deaths in infants.

REFERENCES

KUBLER-ROSS, E. 1976. *On Death and Dying.* Tavistock Publications, London.

MARTINSON, I. 1980. Dying Children at Home. *Nursing Times,* **76**(51), Occasional Paper No. 29, 129–132.

WHALEY, L. F. & WONG, D. L. 1983. *Nursing Care of Infants and Sick Children,* 2nd Edn. Mosby, St Louis.

FURTHER READING

BLUEBOND-LANGNER, M. 1978. *The private worlds of dying children.* Princeton University Press, New Jersey.

BURTON, L. (Ed). 1974. *Care of the child facing death.* Routledge & Kegan Paul, London.

KUBLER-ROSS, E. 1983. *On Children and Death,* Macmillan, London.

SCHIFF, H. S. 1979. *The bereaved parent.* Human Horizons Series. Souvenir Press, London.

11 Paediatric care and the future

In the preceding chapters consideration has been given to paediatric care as it exists now and in the near future. However, as with all areas of nursing it is important to look forward and to prepare ourselves for the changing face of paediatrics.

The World Health Organisation 1986 report *Health For All*, includes the future of children and child care. As a large percentage of the illness in the developing world affects children, we should be thinking about how paediatric nursing can contribute to the vital changes needed to eradicate both complex and simple (e.g. measles) diseases in these countries and to encourage health education.

The European Community Advisory Committee on nurse training (1987) has suggested that there should be a form of reciprocal agreement between European Community member states, for paediatric nurses to practise in each others' countries. However, not all members of the EEC provide a specialist paediatric training, so what effect may this have on standards of care?

Educationally, with the publication of the UKCC (1986) Project 2000, all those caring for children may learn common core topics together and later develop in their area of choice (e.g., paediatric nursing, health visiting and so on). All nurses will have to consider that when children are ill where possible, they should be nursed at home. Greater emphasis will be needed on developing expertise in community paediatric nursing. Resources will determine the number and type of children who can viably be treated in hospital. General management may determine how many and at what level paediatric nurses will be represented in the Health Authority structure.

What sort of problems are likely to increase in the care of children? Whilst technology advances, there is no doubt that more pre-term infants will survive and for longer, that more deformities will be corrected and that genetic engineering may lessen the number of genetically determined diseases.

Research may find out the cause(s) of, for instance, childhood lymphoblastic leukaemia, sudden infant death syndrome and spina bifida. Although prevention of such tragic problems is desirable and the maintenance of human life unquestionable, the moral dilemmas and ethical issues which will arise from life-saving decisions are likely to increase. Legally how much discussion and possible alteration to the law of the land will be needed?

Paediatric nurses are still likely to be faced with treating children from poor socio-economic backgrounds and by children who have been abused.

The effects of the Human Immunodeficiency Viruses (HIV) and the Acquired Immunodeficiency Syndrome (AIDS) have not yet reached their peak in children. What moral conflicts will arise from their consequences can only be conjecture at this stage.

There is no doubt that children will still become ill and require specialist nursing in hospital. The paediatric nurse will need to continue her expertise in areas such as communication, play and observations as well as skills associated with changing technology. Parents will still need comfort, explanation and education. In order to provide the standard of care which sick children require, in the future every nurse should hold a paediatric qualification.

Nursing children is a challenge, requiring a high level of theory and practice, combined with the basic concepts associated with caring. Overall it is an enjoyable experience.

REFERENCES

ADVISORY COMMITTEE ON TRAINING IN NURSING FOR THE EUROPEAN COMMUNITY. 1987. *Report on paediatric training in the European Community.*

UNITED KINGDOM CENTRAL COUNCIL. 1986. *Project 2000: A New Preparation for Practice.* UKCC, London.

WORLD HEALTH ORGANISATION. 1986. *Health for all by the year 2000.* WHO, Geneva.

SOCIETIES AND USEFUL ADDRESSES

Association of British Paediatric Nurses (ABPN)
C/o Central Nursing Office
The Hospital for Sick Children
Great Ormond Street
London, WC1

Foundation for the Study of Infant Deaths
15 Belgrave Square
London, SW1X 8PS

National Association for the Welfare of Children in Hospital (NAWCH)
Argyle House
29–31 Euston Road
London, NW1 2SD

National Society for the Prevention of Cruelty to Children (NSPCC)
1 Riding House Street
London, W1

Royal College of Nursing Paediatric Society
20 Cavendish Square
London, W1M 0AB

Royal Society for the Prevention of Accidents (RoSPA)
Canon House
The Priory
Queensway
Birmingham, B4 6BS

Sickle Cell Society
C/o Brent Community Health Council
Rear Block
16 High Street
Harlesden
London, NW10

The Lisa Sainsbury Foundation
8–10 Crown Hill
Croydon
Surrey, CR0 1RY

The Malcolm Sargent Cancer Fund for Children
56 Redcliffe Square
London, SW10 9HQ

The Spastics Society
12 Park Crescent
London, W1N 4EQ

Voluntary Council for Handicapped Children and
National Children's Bureau
8 Wakely Street
London, EC1V 7QU